BALANCE YOUR ACT

a book for adults with DIABETES

by
Maria Alogna Ludi, BSN, MPH

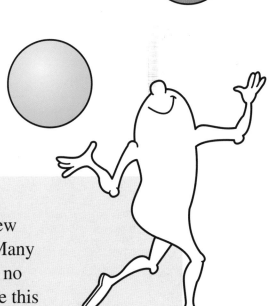

Most people have heard of diabetes, but few know just what it is or how it is treated. Many think that once you have diabetes you can no longer enjoy food, parties or sports. While this is not true, you may feel a loss of freedom. At first diabetes seems to control everything that you do.

How To Use This Book

This book is for all adults with diabetes. On some pages and by some paragraphs, you will see an insulin bottle. This means that what is on that page or in that paragraph is for people with Type 1 diabetes. Much of the information highlighted by the insulin bottles is also for people with Type 2 diabetes who inject insulin. These pages will look like this:

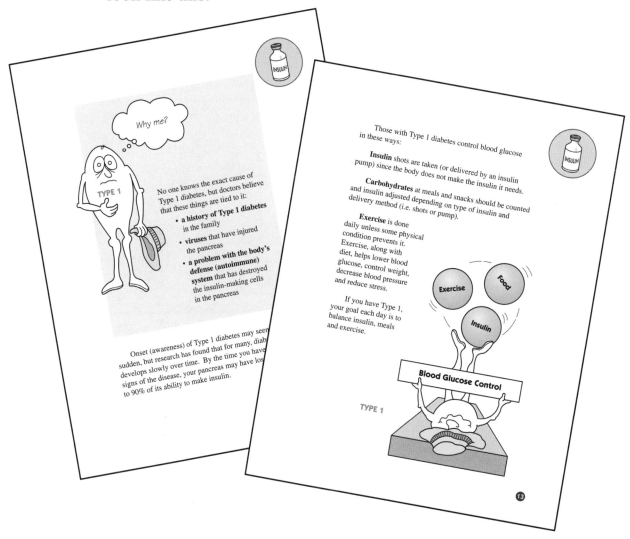

You will also find some blank lines. Some are to be filled in by your doctor or nurse. You may fill in others. This makes the book more personal since everyone's condition and treatment is different.

Table of Contents

Diabetes And The Balancing Act

This book, BALANCE YOUR ACT, helps you gain control of your diabetes and not let it control you. The balance theme refers to the use of foods, activities and medicine for some to control blood glucose. How well you balance what you eat with what you do or take will be your key to a healthy life.

There is a lot to learn about diabetes, and this book is a good place to begin. Use the book as you work with your primary care provider and health care team to learn how to take control of your diabetes.

Share what you learn with your family and friends. They can be helpful and a source of support.

Exercise

Medicines (for some)

Meal Planning

a book for adults with DIABETES

BALANCE YOUR ACT

You have diabetes when the body can't use or make enough insulin. Insulin is a hormone made by the pancreas. This is a gland which sits behind and below the stomach. **Insulin helps get blood glucose** (also called "sugar") **to the cells for energy.** Some glucose also goes to the liver and muscles for storage and future use.

Blood glucose is needed for energy and for brain and nerve functions. A person can't live without it. **Our main source of blood glucose is food.** Foods contain 3 kinds of nutrients: carbohydrates, proteins and fats. All of the carbohydrates, about 50% of the proteins and 10% of the fats from our foods or drinks break down into glucose. As food is eaten, the pancreas sends insulin out into the blood, and insulin gets glucose to the cells for energy.

The American Diabetes Association recommends that people with diabetes maintain blood glucose levels close to the normal range. Blood glucose levels can be checked before or after eating. For adults (men and non-pregnant women), a target blood glucose before eating ranges from 80–120. It may rise after eating but should return to the pre-meal range within 3–4 hours. A target blood glucose at bedtime ranges from 100–140. Your doctor or diabetes educator will tell you what your blood glucose should be—depending on your age and treatment plan.

Write your target blood glucose ranges here:

Before meals _____ to _____

2 hours after meals _____ to _____

Bedtime _____ to _____

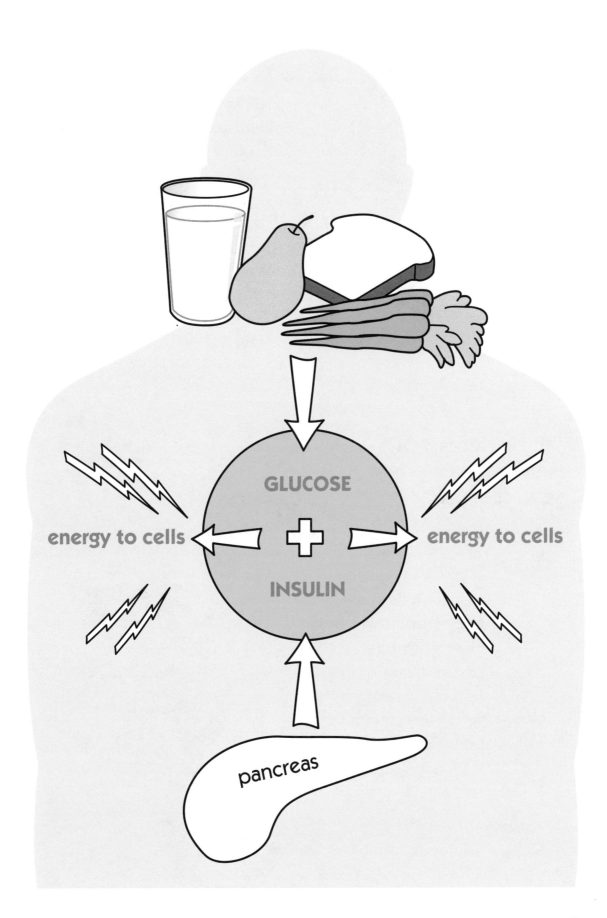

GLUCOSE

+

INSULIN

energy to cells

energy to cells

pancreas

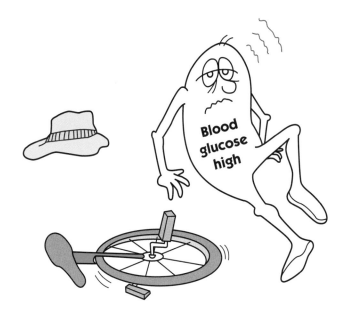

When you have diabetes, glucose builds up in the blood rather than going to the cells. Soon the kidneys can no longer handle this extra glucose, and it spills into the urine and is lost. Since the cells are not getting the glucose they need, you may feel very thirsty, tired or urinate often. You may also lose weight. These are the early signs of high blood glucose (hyperglycemia), but not everyone has them.

With diabetes **YOU** manage your body's use of glucose.

With diabetes, your body can't lower blood glucose on its own. You have to help the body do this. It means learning to balance what you eat with your exercise and any medicines that are prescribed.

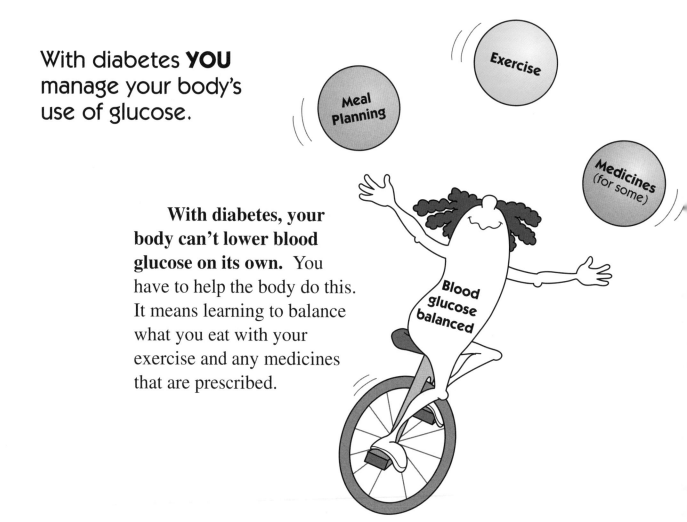

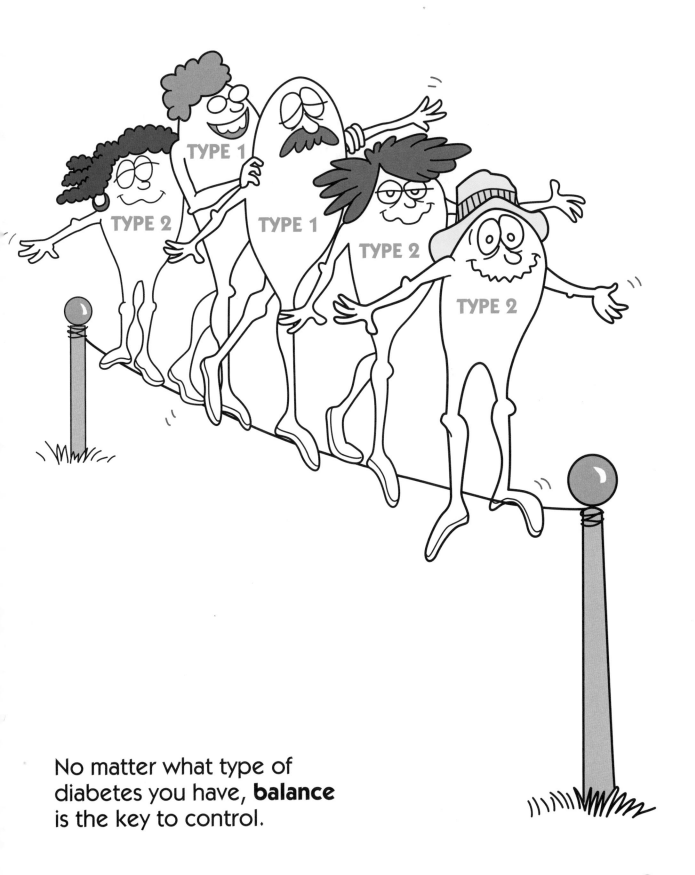

No matter what type of
diabetes you have, **balance**
is the key to control.

Types Of Diabetes

There are four categories of diabetes, and the type depends on what caused it. These four categories are:

- Type 1

- Type 2

- gestational diabetes mellitus (GDM)-
  which occurs during pregnancy

- other specific types (such as those
  caused by medicines and/or other illnesses)

The most common types are Type 1 and Type 2.

Type 1 Diabetes

With Type 1, your body makes little or no insulin. This disease is caused when the beta cells in your pancreas that make insulin are destroyed. People with this kind of diabetes must inject insulin as part of treatment for survival.

Type 1 used to be called *juvenile diabetes* or *insulin-dependent diabetes mellitus* (IDDM). It occurs most often (but not always) in people 30 years old or younger. About 5–10% of all people with diabetes have Type 1.

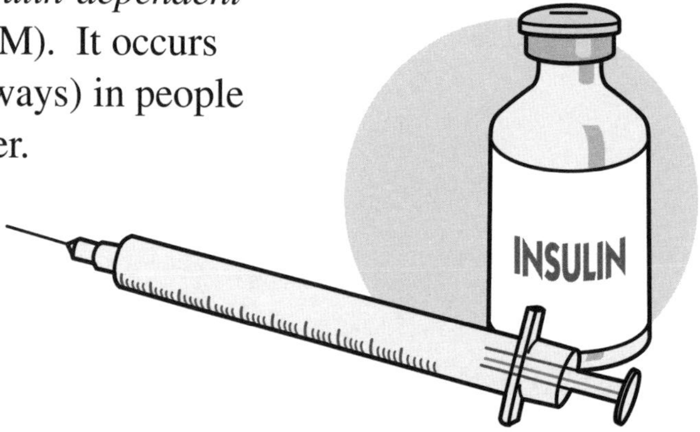

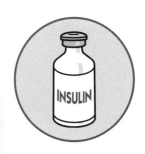

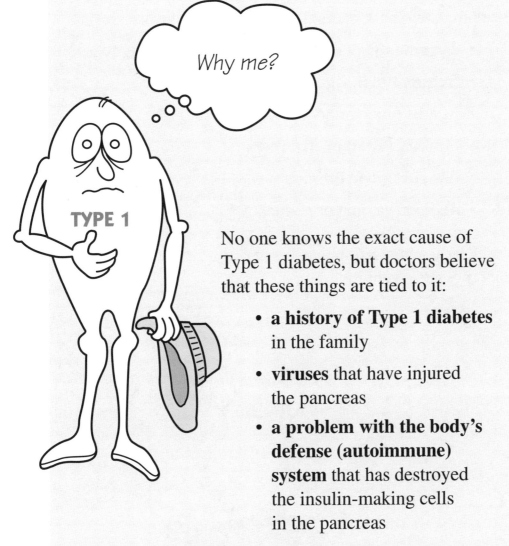

No one knows the exact cause of Type 1 diabetes, but doctors believe that these things are tied to it:

- **a history of Type 1 diabetes** in the family
- **viruses** that have injured the pancreas
- **a problem with the body's defense (autoimmune) system** that has destroyed the insulin-making cells in the pancreas

Onset (awareness) of Type 1 diabetes may seem sudden, but research has found that for many, diabetes develops slowly over time. By the time you have any signs of the disease, your pancreas may have lost up to 90% of its ability to make insulin.

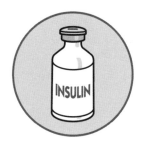

You may have one or more of these symptoms with Type 1 diabetes:

- **extreme thirst or hunger**

- **frequent urination**

- **weight loss** (for no known reason)

- **blurred vision or dizziness**

- **low energy or fatigue**

- **itching** (vaginal or genital)

These symptoms occur when blood glucose is high.

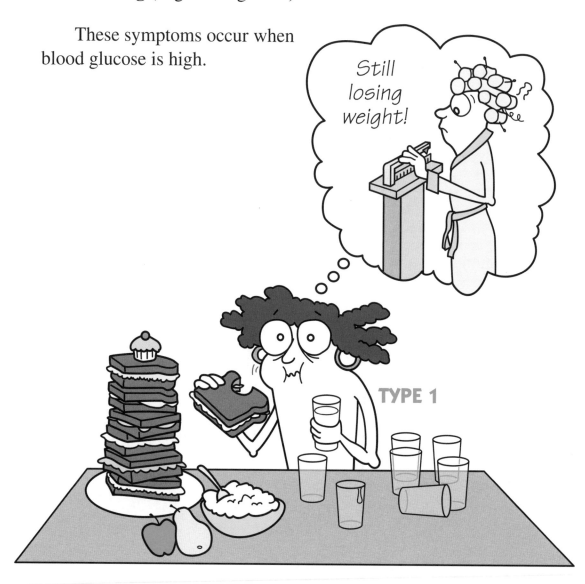

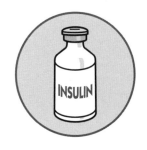

Those with Type 1 diabetes control blood glucose in these ways:

Insulin shots are taken (or delivered by an insulin pump) since the body does not make the insulin it needs.

Carbohydrates at meals and snacks should be counted and insulin adjusted depending on type of insulin and delivery method (i.e. shots or pump).

Exercise is done daily unless some physical condition prevents it. Exercise, along with diet, helps lower blood glucose, control weight, decrease blood pressure and reduce stress.

If you have Type 1, your goal each day is to balance insulin, meals and exercise.

TYPE 1

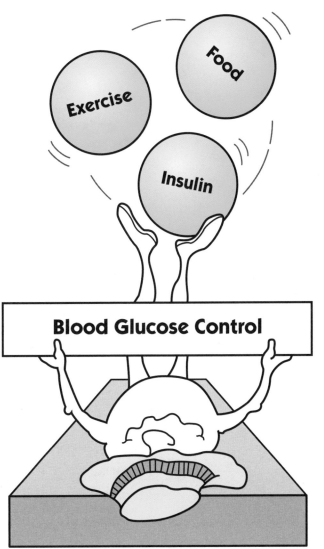

Type 2 Diabetes

This kind of diabetes is caused when the cells in your body can't use insulin as they should and/or your body is making less insulin than it needs. The best way to stay in balance is to manage your diet, exercise and weight. Some people also may need to take oral agents (diabetes pills), inject insulin or do both.

Type 2 diabetes used to be called *adult-onset diabetes* or *non-insulin-dependent diabetes* (NIDDM). This kind of diabetes can develop over a number of years. It may or may not cause severe symptoms. About 90% of people with diabetes have Type 2.

Blood glucose

These factors may lead to Type 2 diabetes:

- **being overweight** Insulin must hook up to *receptors* on the body's cells. It is thought that too much body weight blocks insulin receptor sites. When weight is lost, these receptors become active. Blood glucose improves and can return to normal.

- **family history of diabetes**

- **not being active**
  This can lead to weight gain and cause the body's receptors not to work as they should.

- **ethnic background**
  Your risk may be higher if you are African American, Native American, Hispanic, Asian or Pacific Islander.

Often you feel no symptoms with Type 2 diabetes. Other times, symptoms occur over a period of time or are found on a routine medical checkup. When they occur, you may notice one or more of these:

- **low energy or fatigue**

- **extreme thirst** (dry mouth)

- **blurred vision** or **dizziness**

- **frequent urination**

- **itching** (vaginal or genital)

- **frequent infections** (urinary tract, vaginal, boils, abscesses)

- **weight changes** (gain or loss)

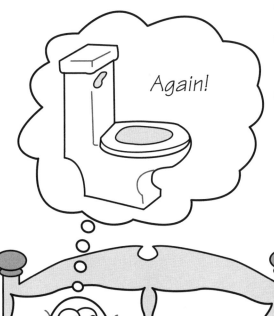

Again!

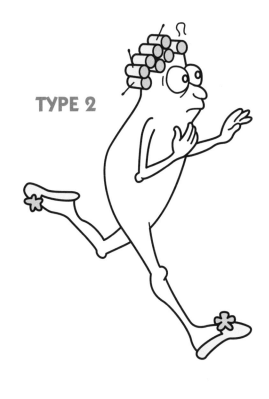

TYPE 2

Most often the treatment for Type 2 diabetes is getting to and staying at a body weight that's right for you (see page 43). Meal planning and exercise can help you lose weight.

If meal planning and exercise are not enough to control blood glucose, an oral diabetes medicine may also be prescribed. These pills (called *oral agents*) help control blood glucose but are **not** insulin. At times, insulin may be required by people with Type 2 diabetes.

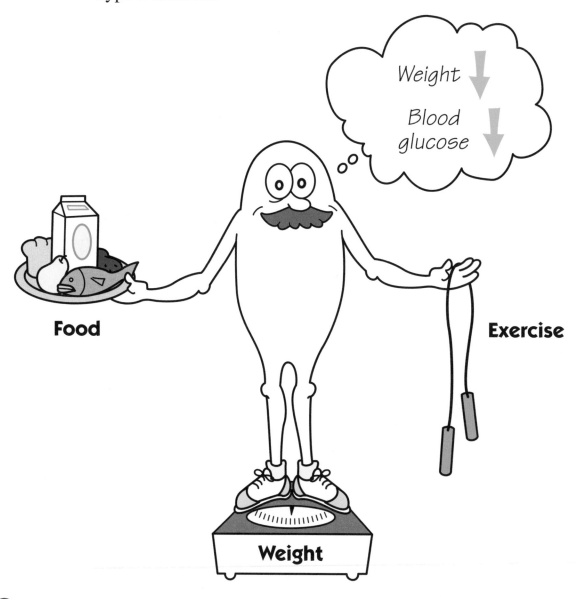

Weight ↓

Blood glucose ↓

Food

Exercise

Weight

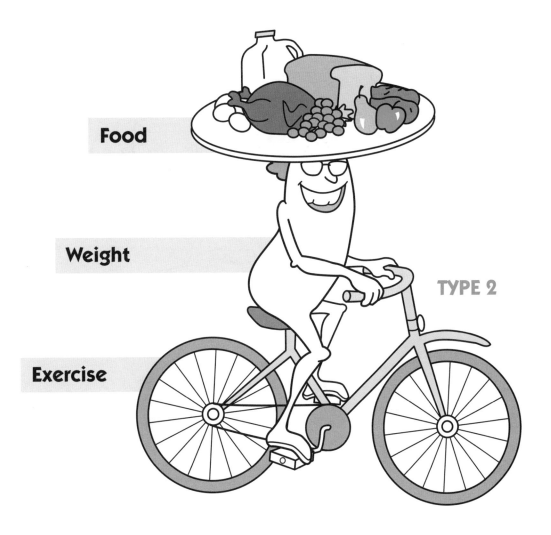

Food

Weight

TYPE 2

Exercise

A **meal plan** is needed and will depend on:

- how much you weigh

- how active you are

- how well your body uses glucose from food

A **healthy body weight** is important because blood glucose is more likely to go down with weight loss. Even a 10 pound weight loss that is kept off can improve your diabetes.

Daily exercise is needed for weight loss and weight control. It also improves cardiovascular function and the way you feel about yourself.

Treatment

The goal in diabetes treatment is to keep your blood glucose as near normal as possible. Extremes either way (high or low) can cause problems.

If blood glucose stays high, you will be prone to problems with circulation and slow-healing infections or injuries. Uncontrolled high blood glucose can cause damage to parts of your body such as the heart and blood vessels, nerves, kidneys, eyes and feet.*

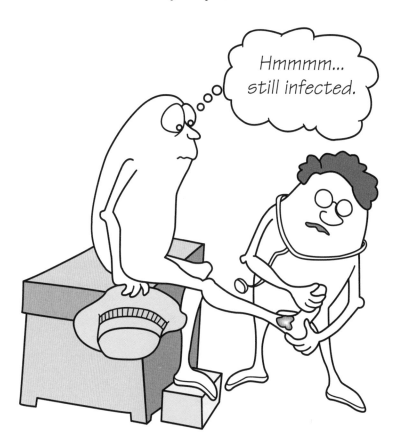

Hmmmm... still infected.

High Blood Glucose

*In 1993, the Diabetes Control and Complications Trial (DCCT) showed that tight control of blood glucose greatly reduces long-term complications for people with Type 1 diabetes. In 1998, the United Kingdom Prospective Diabetes Study (UKPDS) showed similar benefits for people with Type 2 diabetes.

Low blood glucose (hypoglycemia) can cause problems for people taking insulin or pills for diabetes. For example, if you delay or miss a meal or snack, exercise without eating or inject too much insulin, you may feel dizzy or even become unconscious. These extremes (high and low blood glucose) are discussed in detail on pages 65–69.

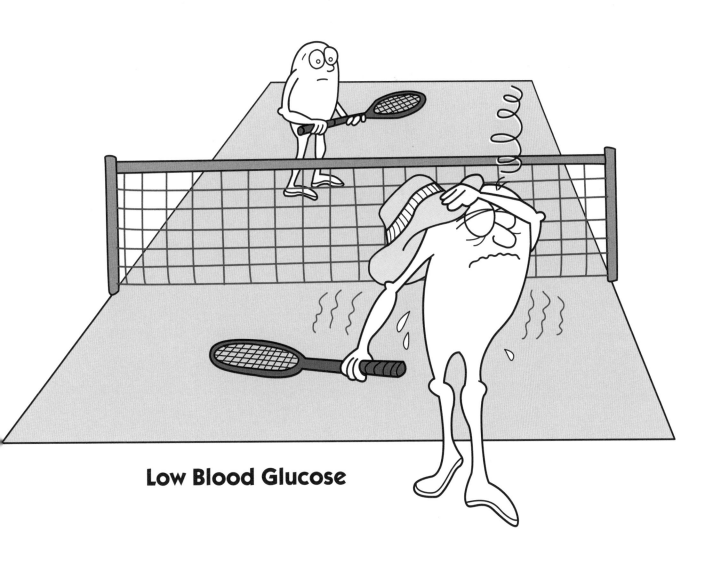

Low Blood Glucose

People with Type 1 diabetes need to inject insulin. Some people with Type 2 diabetes may take a pill to help lower blood glucose. Other times, Type 2's may inject insulin. Sometimes, stress (such as pregnancy, illness or divorce) can cause you to need medicine for a short period of time.

Your goal, to keep as normal a blood glucose as possible, will be reached in one of these ways:

People who have Type 1 diabetes will balance:

- Food

- Exercise

- Insulin

People who have Type 2 diabetes will balance:

- Food

- Exercise

- Body weight

- Oral agents, insulin or both (if needed)

Food

The most important part of treatment is to balance **what** you eat with **how much** and **when** you eat. When you eat the right foods in the right amounts, blood glucose is easier to control.

A registered dietitian can help you and your family plan meals to control blood glucose. What you eat each day depends on how much you weigh, how active you are and which medicines you take.

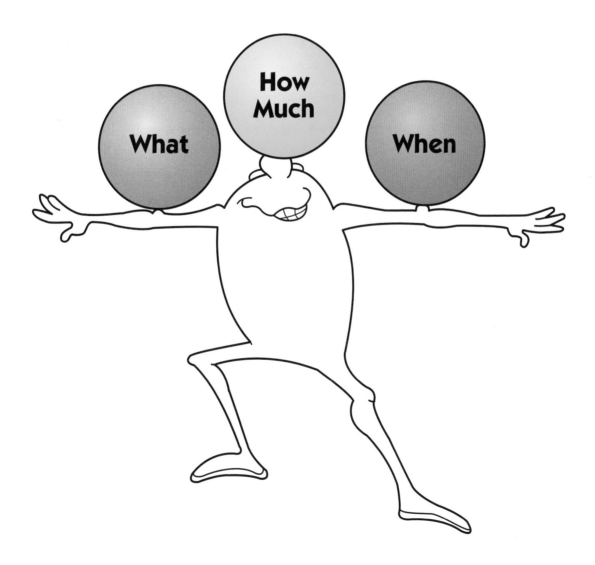

If you take Lantus and rapid acting insulin, count how many carbs you have at meals and take the amount of insulin your doctor or dietitan has chosen for you. If you skip a meal, there is no need to take rapid acting.

Keep these in mind when choosing foods:

If you use insulin:

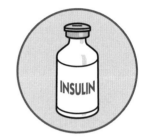

- eat at about the **same times** each day; don't skip or put off meals or snacks

- eat the **right amounts** of the **right foods** at each meal

- eat a **bedtime snack:**
  - if it's part of your meal plan, or
  - if your blood glucose is less than 100

- **eat foods low in fat**

- **exercise some each day**

- **eat before exercising** if blood glucose is less than 100

If you do not use insulin:

- **follow your meal plan** using a variety of healthy foods

- **control portion sizes**

- **balance** the amount of **total carbohydrates** (starch, fruit, milk and sugar) among all your meals

- **eat foods low in sugar, fat and salt**

- **exercise regularly**

- get to a **body weight** that's healthy for you (see page 44) and stay there

Food choices

To help with meal planning, all foods have been put into groups depending on how much carbohydrate, protein and fat they contain. These 3 groups are:

1 *Carbohydrate Group*
Starches
Fruit
Milk
Vegetables
Other Carbohydrates

2 *Protein Group*
Meat and meat substitutes
very lean
lean
medium fat
high fat

3 *Fat Group*
Monounsaturated
Polyunsaturated
Saturated

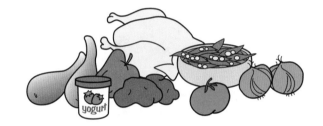

These food groups are called exchanges because you can exchange, or swap, any food in a group for any other food in that group. To order an up-to-date exchange list, call the American Diabetes Association (see page 93).

A registered dietitian can help you work out a meal plan that includes foods you like. There are no "forbidden" foods for a person with diabetes, but there are some you need to be careful about. Having diabetes puts you at risk for heart disease and high blood pressure, so watch your salt intake. You will need to limit the amount and type of fat in your diet. Also, sugar has calories and no vitamins, and many high-sugar foods also have fat.

Eating the right foods in the right amounts will help to control your blood glucose and reduce your risk of other diseases. It will also help you to lose weight if that is one of your treatment goals.

Your dietitian can help you plan what foods to eat using the food pyramid as a guide. For a healthy diet, choose foods from every food group.

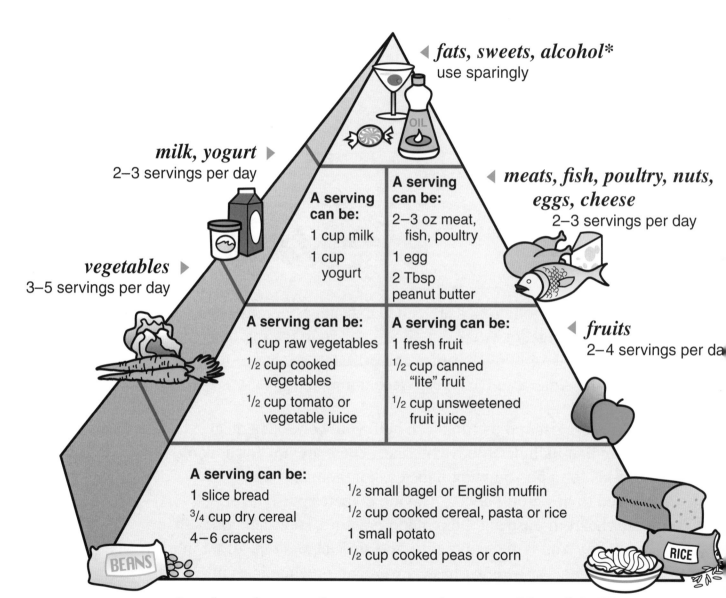

fats, sweets, alcohol*
use sparingly

milk, yogurt ▶
2–3 servings per day

◀ **meats, fish, poultry, nuts, eggs, cheese**
2–3 servings per day

A serving can be:
1 cup milk
1 cup yogurt

A serving can be:
2–3 oz meat, fish, poultry
1 egg
2 Tbsp peanut butter

vegetables ▶
3–5 servings per day

A serving can be:
1 cup raw vegetables
½ cup cooked vegetables
½ cup tomato or vegetable juice

A serving can be:
1 fresh fruit
½ cup canned "lite" fruit
½ cup unsweetened fruit juice

◀ **fruits**
2–4 servings per day

A serving can be:
1 slice bread
¾ cup dry cereal
4–6 crackers
½ small bagel or English muffin
½ cup cooked cereal, pasta or rice
1 small potato
½ cup cooked peas or corn

▲ **grains, breads, cereals, pasta, starchy vegetables, dried beans**
6–11 servings per day

Ask your doctor if you can have alcohol in your diet.

Here's a sample day menu of about 1800 calories:

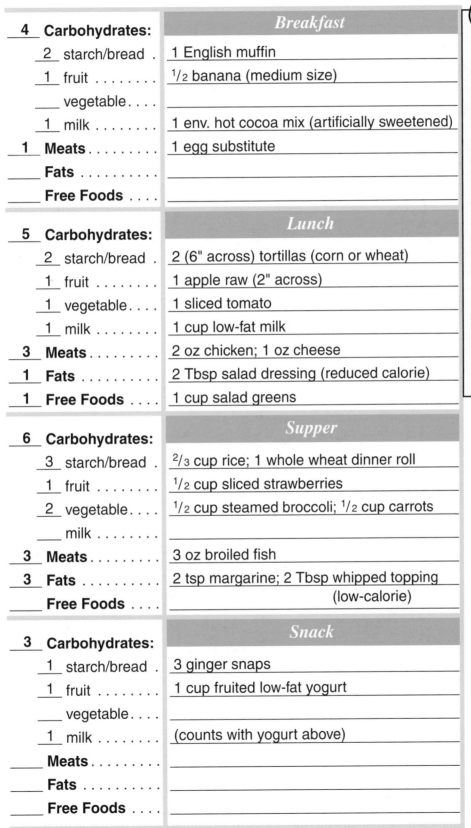

	Breakfast
4 Carbohydrates:	
2 starch/bread .	1 English muffin
1 fruit	½ banana (medium size)
___ vegetable. . . .	
1 milk	1 env. hot cocoa mix (artificially sweetened)
1 Meats	1 egg substitute
___ Fats	
___ Free Foods	

	Lunch
5 Carbohydrates:	
2 starch/bread .	2 (6" across) tortillas (corn or wheat)
1 fruit	1 apple raw (2" across)
1 vegetable. . . .	1 sliced tomato
1 milk	1 cup low-fat milk
3 Meats	2 oz chicken; 1 oz cheese
1 Fats	2 Tbsp salad dressing (reduced calorie)
1 Free Foods	1 cup salad greens

	Supper
6 Carbohydrates:	
3 starch/bread .	⅔ cup rice; 1 whole wheat dinner roll
1 fruit	½ cup sliced strawberries
2 vegetable. . . .	½ cup steamed broccoli; ½ cup carrots
___ milk	
3 Meats	3 oz broiled fish
3 Fats	2 tsp margarine; 2 Tbsp whipped topping
___ Free Foods	(low-calorie)

	Snack
3 Carbohydrates:	
1 starch/bread .	3 ginger snaps
1 fruit	1 cup fruited low-fat yogurt
___ vegetable. . . .	
1 milk	(counts with yogurt above)
___ Meats	
___ Fats	
___ Free Foods	

Carbohydrate choices can be made from starches/breads, fruits and milk. You do not have to count the carbohydrates in 1 or 2 servings of vegetables because they have only small amounts. Try to eat 1–2 vegetable servings at lunch and supper. Check your exchange list.

Measuring foods for exact amounts

Portion size is very important. You may want to use a **measuring cup, measuring spoons** and **small scale** to get used to what 2 oz of meat or ½ cup of cooked peas looks like when served. Measure meats **after they are cooked and trimmed of fat.** Also be sure to measure fats such as margarine, mayonnaise and cooking oils with care.

If you are taking insulin, you need to balance your insulin, food and exercise. To do this, you need to be consistent with these. This means:

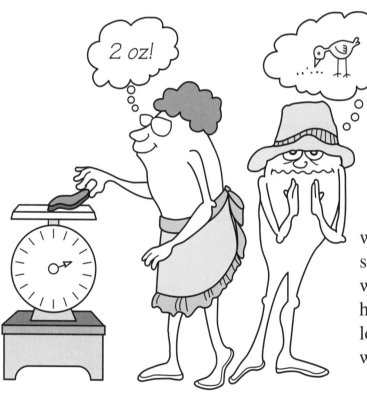

- eat a set amount of carbohydrate at each meal and snack

- do not skip meals

- exercise and inject insulin at the same times each day

People trying to manage their weight need to control portion sizes. This is true for those who want to lose weight or maintain a healthy body weight. As you start losing weight, your insulin doses will need to be adjusted.

NOTE: If you are taking insulin or pills for diabetes, delaying or skipping a meal can cause low blood glucose. Skipping a meal can cause you to eat more at the next meal. Besides making it harder to "do your balancing act," this can also make it harder to lose weight.

Seasonings & free foods

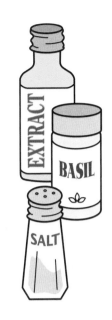

When you look at your ADA Exchange List, you will see that some foods and seasonings may be eaten and not be counted as exchanges. These are called "free foods," and they have less than 20 calories or less than 5 grams of carbohydrate per serving. You can eat as much as you want of these foods when no serving size is given. If a serving size is listed, you can eat up to 3 servings a day of free foods. Spread these out over a number of meals and snacks each day. Eating all 3 servings at one time could affect your blood glucose level.

fat-free/reduced-fat

1 Tbsp cream cheese, fat-free
1 Tbsp nondairy creamer (liquid)
1 Tbsp nondairy creamer (powder)
1 Tbsp mayonnaise, fat-free
1 tsp mayonnaise, reduced-fat
4 Tbsp margarine, fat-free
1 tsp margarine, reduced-fat
1 Tbsp Miracle Whip, fat-free
1 tsp Miracle Whip, reduced-fat
nonstick cooking spray
1 Tbsp salad dressing, fat-free
2 Tbsp Italian salad dressing, fat-free
¼ cup salsa
1 Tbsp sour cream, fat-free or reduced-fat
2 Tbsp whipped topping, regular or light

sugar-free/low-sugar

1 hard candy, sugar-free
2 tsp jam or jelly, low sugar or light
sugar-free gelatins
sugar-free gum
sugar substitutes
2 Tbsp syrup, sugar-free

drinks

bouillon, broth, consomme*
1 Tbsp cocoa powder, unsweetened
coffee
sugar-free soft drinks
sugar-free drink mixes
tea

condiments

1 Tbsp catsup
1½ large dill pickles*
horseradish
lemon & lime juice
mustard
soy sauce*
1 Tbsp taco sauce
vinegar

seasonings

garlic
herbs, fresh or dried
pimiento
spices
Tabasco or hot pepper sauce
vanilla or other extracts
wine used in cooking
Worcestershire sauce

These may not be allowed for those on low-sodium diets.

Carbohydrates

When you have diabetes, carbohydrate is the most important nutrient to understand. It breaks down almost 100% into blood glucose within 1½ hours after eating it.

Sugar and starch are carbohydrates, and there are 2 kinds—**complex** and **simple**. **Complex carbohydrate** is found in starchy foods like bread, pasta, corn, beans, peas and potatoes. Fruits have **simple carbohydrate** but also are high in fiber and vitamins and low in fat.

Foods like cake, ice cream and chocolate contain sugar (also a **simple carbohydrate**). They also have a lot of fat. **Simple carbohydrates** like jelly and honey are not high-fat but have a lot of calories and no vitamins or minerals.

Having diabetes does not mean that you can't eat sweets. It does mean you have to be careful to decide how much you can have and what you might have to omit from the other parts of the meal. Light desserts can be made with fruits (fresh, frozen or canned in light syrup or without sugar added) and/or artificial sweeteners and be counted as carbohydrate in your meal plan. These are some examples:

- frozen yogurt, low-fat ice cream
- gingersnaps, graham crackers, vanilla wafers
- sugar-free pudding

Sugar (sucrose) and foods sweetened with sugar also can be planned into your diet with the help of a dietitian. These foods must be exchanged for the carbohydrate foods in your meal plan—not added as an extra. Extra food choices may lead to weight gain and poor blood glucose control. (See page 91 for cookbooks that can help.)

Carbohydrate Counting

Another approach to meal planning with diabetes is carbohydrate counting. Ask your dietitian if this would work for you.

Carbohydrate (carb) counting is a way to control the amount of carbs (sugars and starches) you eat. Counting the grams of carbs you eat will help you have the recommended number of carbs each day. If you take insulin, this can help you take the right amount of insulin for what and how much you eat.

Calories from all foods, including fats and protein, are changed into glucose, but not as fast as carbohydrates. Carbs are changed into glucose within an hour after a meal. So, you need to know the number of carbs you eat at each meal to control your blood glucose levels.

As a rule, 50-60% of your total calories for the day should come from carbohydrates. They should be spread among your meals and snacks depending on your needs, medication and lifestyle.

For each meal and snack, you should know the number of grams of carbs your doctor or dietitian has set for you and the amount of carbs in different foods. The amount of carbs in a food can be found on its food label.

While counting carbs in different foods, keep in mind that even though foods may have the same amount of carbs, one may have more fat than another. These added calories can lead to weight gain. This is really important for foods made with added sugar like candy, cookies, cakes or other desserts. Even though you can include these desserts in your meal plan with carb counting, the goal is still to eat healthy foods.

Using carb counting can help you feel more "in control" whether you use insulin or diet alone to control diabetes. Taking control of your diet will lead to good control of your blood glucose and your diabetes. The more you know about this, the more freedom you can have in managing your diabetes.

Spread your carbs out over the day

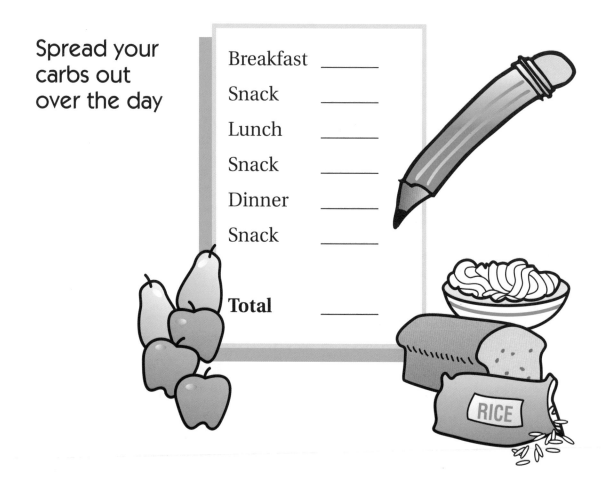

Breakfast _____

Snack _____

Lunch _____

Snack _____

Dinner _____

Snack _____

Total _____

Food labels

Reading food labels can help promote healthy eating habits. To know what is really in a food, keep these in mind when reading the **Nutrition Facts** on a food label*:

- The **serving size** on the label may not be the serving size on the exchange list. You may need to adjust the serving size.

- The **Total Carbohydrate** listing is important to people with diabetes. Your body breaks down the carbohydrate in food into blood glucose.

- **Sugars are part of the Total Carbohydrate** listed on the label. The sugars listed on food labels can be added sugars or sugars that occur naturally.

- Fiber is also part of **Total Carbohydrate.**

- Be aware of the grams of **Total Fat** in one serving. One fat choice from the exchange list has 5 grams of fat.

- Limit **Saturated Fat** to no more than 10% of all calories eaten. This type of fat raises cholesterol.

Some labels are too small to have Nutrition Facts. By law, these labels must have a phone number or address for you to get this information.

Nutrition Facts

Serving Size 9.0 oz (240 grams)
Servings Per Container 1

Amount Per Serving

Calories 250   Calories from Fat 18

% Daily Value*

Total Fat 2g	**3**%
Saturated Fat Less than 1 g	**5**%
Cholesterol 20 mg	**7**%
Sodium 420 mg	**18**%
Total Carbohydrate 44g	**15**%
Dietary Fiber 2g	**8**%
Sugars 4g	
Protein 14g	

Vitamin A	50%	•	Vitamin C	8%
Calcium	25%	•	Iron	15%

* Percent Daily Values are based on a 2,000 calorie diet. Your daily values may be higher or lower depending on your calorie needs:

	Calories	2,000	2,500
Total Fat	Less than	65g	80g
Sat Fat	Less than	20g	25g
Cholesterol	Less than	300mg	300mg
Sodium	Less than	2,400mg	2,400mg
Total Carbohydrate		300g	375g
Dietary Fiber		25g	30g

Calories per gram:
Fat 9   •   Carbohydrates 4   •   Protein 4

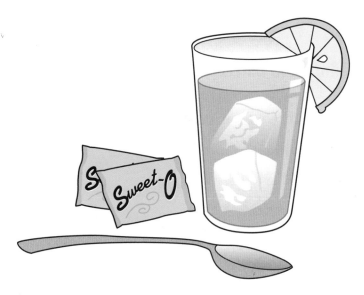

Artificial sweeteners

Aspartame and saccharin are 2 common artificial sweeteners. They are in many products which you can use. They are both approved by the Food and Drug Administration (FDA).

Aspartame is 200 times sweeter than sugar, and you can use very little to get a lot of sweetness. You can buy it in packets or tablets for use in drinks or foods. One packet or two tablets is the same as 2 teaspoons of sugar.

Check the labels on sweeteners to see if they contain aspartame or saccharin.

There are also newer artificial sweeteners on the market. One is called acesulfame K (Sunett). This sweetener is not harmed by heat and can be used in cooking. Another is Splenda, a product made with sucralose. It has no calories and no effect on blood glucose of HbA1c. Both of these are also approved by the FDA. You may want to ask your doctor or nutritionist about using these.

Dietetic foods

Dietetic foods made with fructose, xylitol, mannitol or sorbitol have calories and carbohydrate. **(Large amounts** of zylitol, mannitol or sorbitol **can cause diarrhea.)** Many times a dietetic product has as many calories as the food it is trying to copy. For those who need to lose weight, these products will be of **no benefit**. (Often you may find these foods cost more and do not taste like the food they copy.) Foods like these must be counted in a meal plan just like any other food.

Some foods labeled "dietetic" may be low in sugar but still be high in total carbohydrate, fat, cholesterol or sodium. Some low-fat foods may be higher in carbohydrate and sodium than the regular product. Read labels with care. Foods labeled sugar-free may not have sugar but will have other sweeteners high in carbohydrates and calories.

Fiber

Dietary fiber is the part of plant foods that is not digested. There are 2 types, soluble and insoluble fiber. Foods high in soluble fiber may help reduce fatty buildup in the arteries (atherosclerosis). Some good sources are:

- dried beans, peas, lentils

- whole fruit

- oat bran, barley, bulgar

Foods high in insoluble fiber help prevent constipation and may help reduce the risk of colon cancer and other digestive problems. Some good sources are:

- wheat bran
- most grains

- vegetables
- nuts

Cholesterol & saturated fats

Foods high in cholesterol and saturated fat promote fatty buildup in the arteries (atherosclerosis). Having diabetes also makes you prone to fatty buildup. As more fat clogs the arteries, the heart pumps harder to send blood through the narrowed vessels.

Most food choices on an Exchange List are already low in cholesterol and saturated fat. Eating these foods, along with regular exercise, may help you prevent heart disease or a heart attack. Your doctor may ask you to eat lean meats or fish and low-fat or fat free dairy foods. Also limit greasy or fried foods and eat no more than 3 or 4 egg yolks a week.

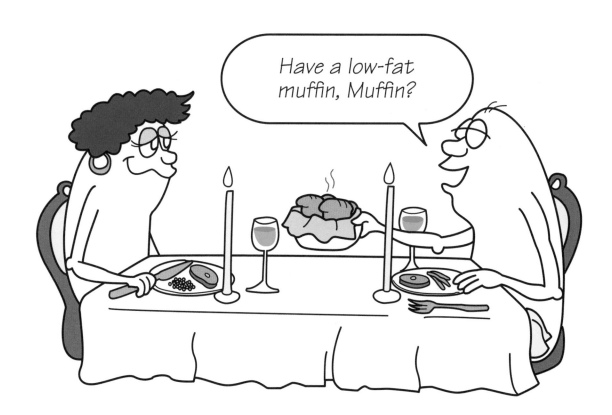

Eating out

Ask yourself these questions when eating out:

- **What will I be served and at what hour?** (To avoid delays, try to make a reservation.) If you think you will be eating later than usual, eat a snack such as fruit before going out. Or, before a late dinner, you could eat your bedtime snack at the normal meal time. Discuss with your doctor or certified diabetes educator when you should take your insulin or medication for these special events.

- **How many exchanges or carbohydrate choices are in the meal?** Until you get used to your diet, carry along an exchange list to be sure of portion sizes. If you can't tell what is in a dish, ask. If you do not think you can get fresh fruit, take some with you.

It is always best to **order broiled**, **baked** or **steamed** foods. Choose foods listed on the menu as "heart healthy." Ask for any dressings to be served on the side. Avoid casseroles or foods with sauces or breading because you may be getting much more carbohydrate and fat than you think.

Here are some tips for when you must choose from "fast foods." Order:

- grilled or baked (such as chicken)

- no mayo, cheese or extra sauces

- light or lean choices advertised to have lower fat

If you are trying to lose weight, think about these when eating out:

- Order **broiled, baked** or **steamed** foods and fresh vegetables, fruits and salads. Pass up the fried foods, butter, gravy, cream sauces and heavy salad dressings.

- Carry a copy of your meal plan along, and **stay within your portion sizes.** You can always take the extra home.

- **Avoid "all you can eat" restaurants or buffets.** (Even at a salad bar, calories add up quickly if you choose things like eggs, cheese and high-fat dressings.)

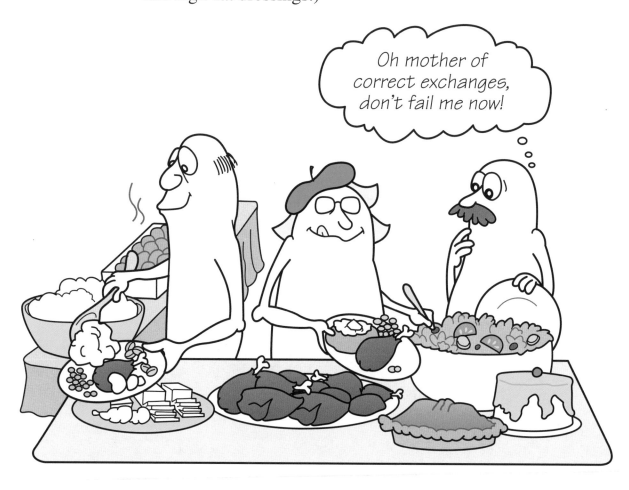

Oh mother of correct exchanges, don't fail me now!

Exercise

Exercise is a major part of treatment for diabetes. What exercise does for you depends on what kind you do, how often you do it and for how long. **Check with your doctor before starting any exercise program.** Here is what exercise can do for people with diabetes:

- **help the body use insulin better**
- **lower blood glucose**
- **burn calories** (weight control)
- **improve muscle tone and heart function**
- **improve sense of well-being**

People with diabetes should have a complete medical exam before starting to exercise. You should not exercise when your blood glucose is very high (240+) or if urine ketones are present. (You can also check for ketones in your blood with a meter.) Contact your doctor if your blood glucose stays high or if you check your urine for ketones and they are moderate or large.

Many people with diabetes will be told to exercise in a group with medical supervision. Your doctor or exercise specialist will tell you what type of exercise to do and how hard to work out.

Counting calories is one way of deciding how much exercise to do. Here is a sample of some exercises and the number of calories they burn:

Activity	Calories burned per hour
Walk	250–450
Swim, jog, cycle	400–650
Climb stairs, skip rope, cross-country ski machine	more than 400

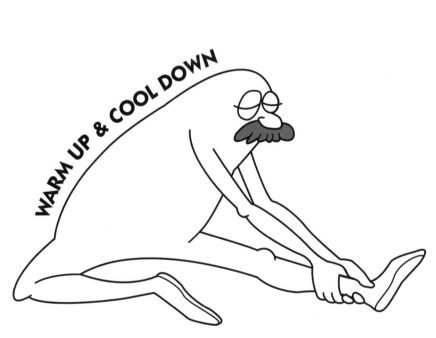

WARM UP & COOL DOWN

Here are some other points to keep in mind about exercise:

- **Warm up before exercise, and cool down afterwards.** Walk slowly for 5–10 minutes to warm up. Then stretch your muscles before going on to harder exercise. This helps loosen the muscles to prevent injuries. Slow walking and stretching after hard exercise help the heart adjust to a slower beat and keep muscles from cramping.

- **Exercise each day in some way.** Use the stairs instead of elevators or escalators. Walk to nearby stores. Take a short walk during a work break.

- **Start slowly and set a pace that is right for you.** For one person, exercise with an easy home-walk program might look like this:

week 1–2	walk ¼ mile (once a day)	5 min.
week 3	walk ¼ mile (twice a day)	5 min. each time

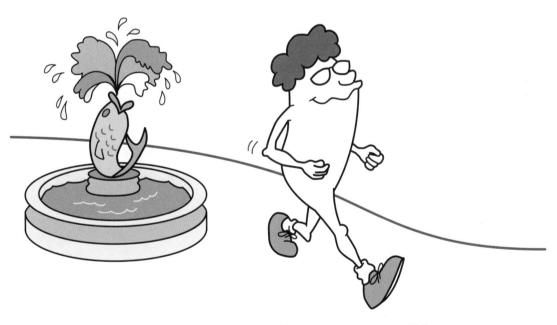

In bad weather, you can keep up your walking exercise at an enclosed mall. Walking is a cheap and safe way to exercise.

Your doctor will tell you what pace to follow for any type of exercise. (Those with foot or leg problems may need to find other ways to exercise safely.)

- Wear shoes that **support** your feet well, and wear **comfortable** clothes.

- **If playing a team sport or joining a dance or exercise class,** make sure the coach or teacher knows that you are on insulin or an oral agent. He or she will need to know the symptoms of low blood glucose and how to treat them. (See pages 65–67.)

- **Do not inject insulin into areas which will be used in exercise.** If jogging, dancing, playing tennis or playing touch football, inject insulin in the abdomen rather than arms or legs. Exercise can speed up the use of insulin from an arm or leg site.

- **Take change with you** so you can call for help if you need it. Or, if you have a cell phone, carry it with you.

- **Always carry some form of treatment.**

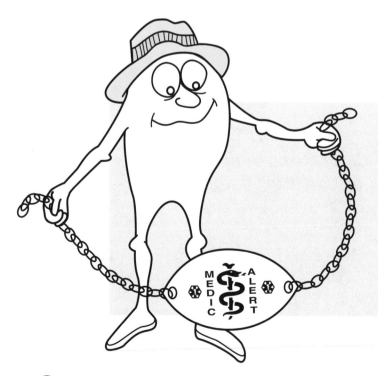

- **Always wear identification (ID).** If you have an accident or pass out, an ID bracelet or necklace tells others that you have diabetes. (See page 83 for Medic Alert ID.)

Exercise precautions

(for those who inject insulin or take oral agents that can cause low blood glucose)

During exercise, your body uses insulin and blood glucose faster. So you must know your blood glucose level and how to adjust foods and insulin to suit your workout. Here are some guides:

- Always **check your blood glucose before and after** exercise.

- **If you are taking insulin or pills** that can cause low blood glucose, check your blood glucose before exercise. If it is not at least 100, have a snack with carbohydrates **before you exercise.**

- To avoid low blood glucose reactions, **do not exercise when insulin is at its peak.**

- **Carry a sugar source with you** when you exercise (like glucose tablets—see page 66).

- **If you often have low blood glucose reactions with exercise, tell your doctor.** It may be wise to exercise with a friend.

- **When blood glucose is close to normal, eat before exercising.** If you don't, blood glucose may drop too low during exercise.

- **You may want to talk with your doctor or diabetes educator** about how to adjust your insulin for exercising.

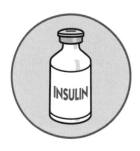

- **If blood glucose is very high** (240+) **or ketones are present** in a urine test, **do not exercise.** Wait until blood glucose comes down because exercise at this time can raise blood glucose even higher. Contact your doctor if your blood glucose stays high or if urine ketones are moderate to large. (As a rule, urine ketone testing is done by people with Type 1 diabetes or lean people with Type 2 diabetes who take insulin.)

- **If you plan to exercise an area of your body where you normally inject insulin, use a different injection site before that exercise.** (For example, if you plan to run, inject your abdomen instead of your leg.)

- **Wear shoes and socks that fit well and protect your feet. Check your feet after exercise** and report any problems (like blisters or infections) to your doctor.

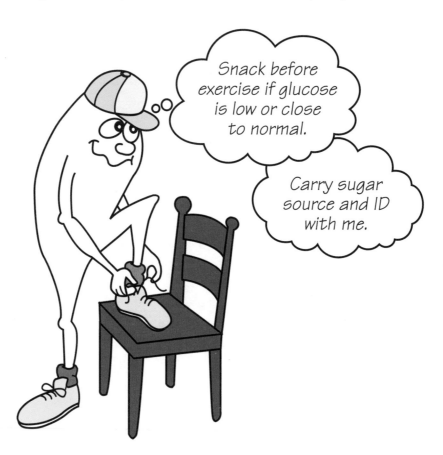

Weight

Weight control is important for anyone with diabetes. Your body makes and/or uses insulin best when you are at or closer to a weight that's right for you. And with better use of insulin, blood glucose comes down. For most people with Type 2 diabetes, weight control and exercise are the primary ways to improve blood glucose.

Meal planning plus exercise helps you control weight. As you start to balance what you eat with how active you are, you are likely to see your weight change. If you eat less than your body needs for activities, you will lose weight. If you eat more than your body needs, you will gain weight.

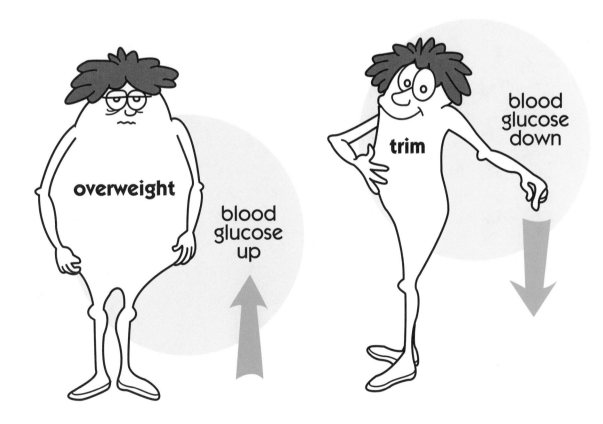

overweight

blood glucose up

trim

blood glucose down

Ask your doctor or dietitian to help you set a good weight goal. If you lose slowly (no more than 1-2 pounds a week) you are more likely to keep it off.

Body mass index (BMI)*

Use this body mass index (BMI) chart to tell if you are overweight. If your BMI score is **24 or less,** you are at a **healthy weight.** If your BMI score is **25 to 29.9,** you are **overweight.** If your BMI score is **30 or more,** you are considered **obese.**

To use the BMI chart, find your height in inches on the left side of the chart (Example: 5 feet = 60 inches). Then move across that row until you find your weight. Now, look at the number at the top of your weight column. That is your BMI score.

Your BMI score is:																
19	20	21	22	23	24	25	26	27	28	29	30	31	32	33	34	35
Your Weight (pounds)																
58"	91	96	100	105	110	115	119	124	129	134	138	143	148	153	158	162	167
59"	94	99	104	109	114	119	124	128	133	138	143	148	153	158	163	168	173
60"	97	102	107	112	118	123	128	133	138	143	148	153	158	163	168	174	179
61"	100	106	111	116	122	127	132	137	143	148	153	158	164	169	174	180	185
62"	104	109	115	120	126	131	136	142	147	153	158	164	169	175	180	186	191
63"	107	113	118	124	130	135	141	146	152	158	163	169	175	180	186	191	197
64"	110	116	122	128	134	140	145	151	157	163	169	174	180	186	192	197	204
65"	114	120	126	132	138	144	150	156	162	168	174	180	186	192	198	204	210
66"	118	124	130	136	142	148	155	161	167	173	179	186	192	198	204	210	216
67"	121	127	134	140	146	153	159	166	172	178	185	191	198	204	211	217	223
68"	125	131	138	144	151	158	164	171	177	184	190	197	203	210	216	223	230
69"	128	135	142	149	155	162	169	176	182	189	196	203	209	216	223	230	236
70"	132	139	146	153	160	167	174	181	188	195	202	209	216	222	229	236	243
71"	136	143	150	157	165	172	179	186	193	200	208	215	222	229	236	243	250
72"	140	147	154	162	169	177	184	191	199	206	213	221	228	235	242	250	258
73"	144	151	159	166	174	182	189	197	204	212	219	227	235	242	250	257	265
74"	148	155	163	171	179	186	194	202	210	218	225	233	241	249	256	264	272
75"	152	160	168	176	184	192	200	208	216	224	232	240	248	256	264	272	279
76"	156	164	172	180	189	197	205	213	221	230	238	246	254	263	271	279	287

Your Height (inches)

* from the National Heart, Lung and Blood Institute

Insulin

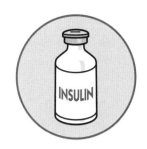

Insulin must be taken by injection. There are several methods that can be used to inject insulin (like a syringe, insulin pen or pump). Your doctor can tell you the best way for you to do this. **Insulin cannot be taken by mouth.** Stomach juices would destroy it before it could be used.

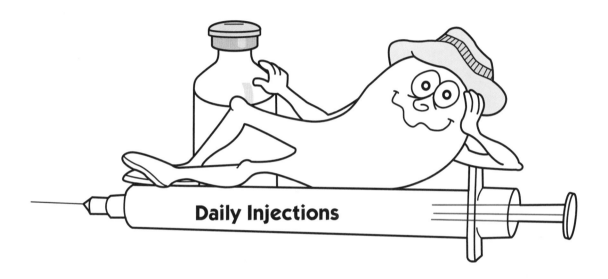

Daily Injections

There are a number of types of insulin. The main things that make them different are:

- **when they begin to act**
- **when they peak**
- **how long they last**

How one person responds to a type of insulin differs from another. Your doctor will work with you to find the type(s) and amount of insulin you need.

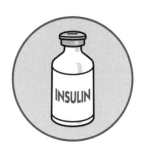

When insulins act & how long

Like any medicine, insulin takes a certain amount of time to begin working. This is called the **onset of action.** After onset, insulin reaches its full effect or **peak action.** From its peak, insulin lasts a fairly short time before it is used up by the body and more is needed. This is called **length of action.**

So to control diabetes 24 hours a day, you may need to take 2 types of insulin with different length and peak actions. These insulins can often be combined in one syringe. Check with your doctor or diabetes educator before mixing insulins. For many people with diabetes, the best way to reach their goals for blood glucose control is to divide the insulin into 2 or more injections a day. Insulin needs to be taken about the same times each day.

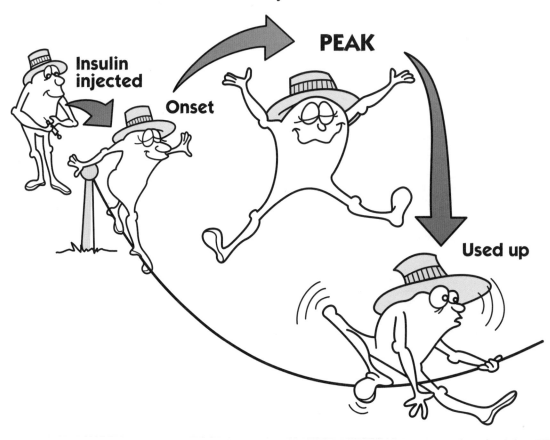

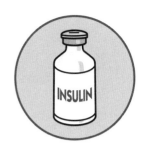

The onset, peak and length of action depend on many things: the type of insulin; your activity level; and where on your body you inject the insulin.

Your doctor will prescribe:

- the type and brand of insulin you will take

- how often and at what times to take it

- the dose

- if it will be more than one type or a premixed type

Write in these facts about your insulin:

Time I take it: _____

Type of insulin: _____

Begins to work _____ hour(s) after injecting.

Peak action _____ hours after injecting.

Lasts _____ hours.

Time I take it: _____

Type of insulin: _____

Begins to work _____ hour(s) after injecting.

Peak action _____ hours after injecting.

Lasts _____ hours.

Time I take it: _____

Type of insulin: _____

Begins to work _____ hour(s) after injecting.

Peak action _____ hours after injecting.

Lasts _____ hours.

Time I take it: _____

Type of insulin: _____

Begins to work _____ hour(s) after injecting.

Peak action _____ hours after injecting.

Lasts _____ hours.

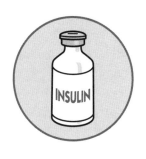

Storing insulin

Always keep one or more extra bottles of insulin on hand at home or on trips.

When traveling, keep insulin and syringes with you at all times. For easy travel, ask your doctor or diabetes educator about a diabetes pen. Any form of insulin will fit in a pocket or purse, but never leave insulin where it is very hot (more than 86°F) or below freezing. (For example, **don't store** in the glove compartment of your car or **directly on ice** in an ice chest.) You can use a Thermos-type jar, or you may want to buy a special storage container.

These facts about storage apply to most insulins. **Check with your doctor and pharmacist** about how best to store yours.

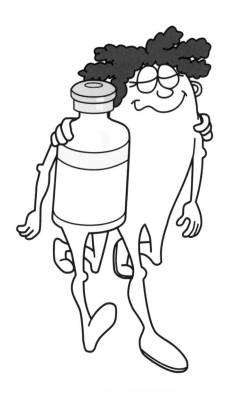

- Keep unopened insulin in the refrigerator, but **do not freeze.**

- Once opened, insulin may be stored in the refrigerator (for longer life) or at room temperature. (Keep out of direct sunlight and **discard after 30 days.**)

- Whether you store opened insulin in the refrigerator or not, **do not use after expiration date** on bottle.

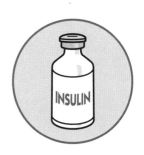

Syringes

Syringes can be bought at any drugstore, but you may need a prescription. They can be bought in several sizes. Some can hold 100 units of insulin. Others can hold only 30 or 50 units of insulin. They are marked in units by little lines like a ruler.

Check with your doctor or diabetes educator to see which size insulin syringe works best for you. Also check to see what needle length is right for you. There are very short needles and regular needles available for syringes and pens.

U-100 Insulin Syringe

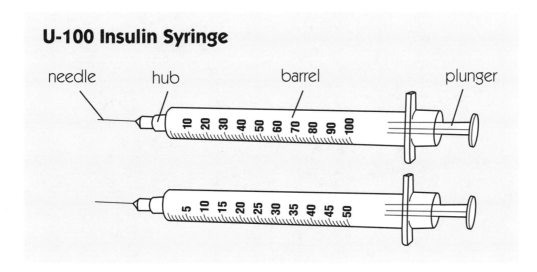

needle   hub   barrel   plunger

Used Sharps (syringes and lancets)*

Used sharps should be treated as medical waste. If you do not dispose of your syringes safely, it puts people at risk and you can be fined. Your community may have a special program for safely collecting medical waste. If not, you will need to buy a sharps container at a drugstore or medical supply store. Call your sanitation or county health department to learn the state or county laws you must follow.

*Ask your doctor or diabetes educator about reusing syringes.

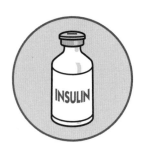

Injection sites

There are a number of places (sites) on the body where you may inject insulin. These places have enough fatty tissue to absorb it. The abdomen is thought to be the best place.

Where you inject insulin affects how fast it is absorbed. Exercise can speed up the use of insulin from an arm or leg site, so always use your abdomen if you plan to exercise soon after taking your shot.

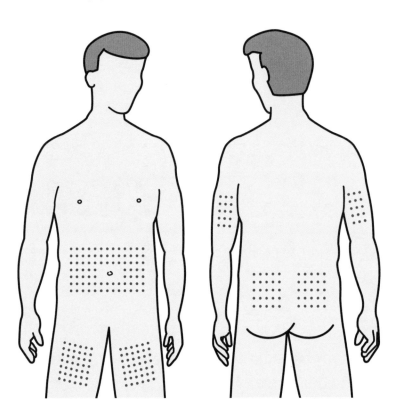

Decide with your doctor or diabetes educator which areas of the body are best for you. You can rotate sites within one area for one week at a time. Keep injection sites within the area at least one inch apart. Some people use abdomen sites most of the time by moving at least an inch from the last injection.

How to draw up insulin

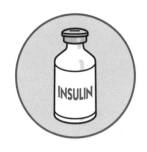

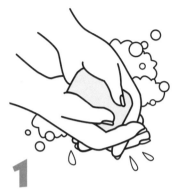

1
Wash your hands.

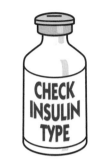

2
Check bottle label to make sure it is the right insulin.

3
Check expiration date. Do not use expired insulin.

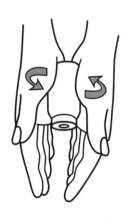

4
Roll insulin between hands to mix well. (Cloudy insulin must be rolled to mix.)

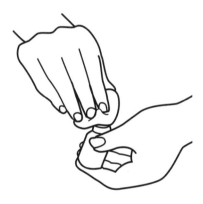

5
Wipe top of insulin bottle with alcohol.

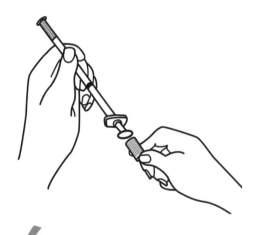

6
Take syringe out of package and remove plastic from plunger.

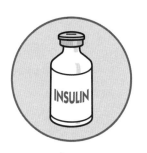

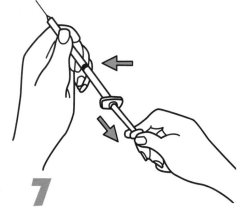

7

Remove cap from needle. (**Never** touch needle with your hands.) Pull plunger down to number of units of insulin needed (for example, 20 units). You are filling syringe with air.

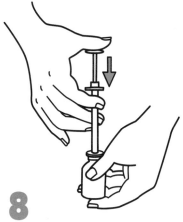

8

With plunger out, push needle into bottle. Then push plunger in. This injects air into bottle. (If you don't inject air, a vacuum occurs that makes it hard to pull insulin out of the bottle.)

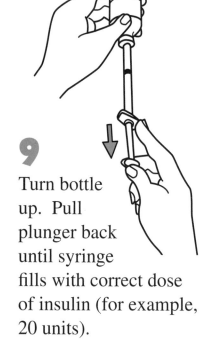

9

Turn bottle up. Pull plunger back until syringe fills with correct dose of insulin (for example, 20 units).

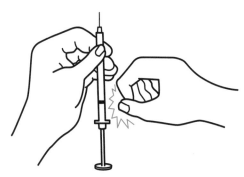

10

Remove syringe from bottle. Check insulin in syringe for bubbles. If there are air bubbles, tap syringe until bubbles are all at the top. Push the plunger to get them out. (They won't hurt you, but bubbles may keep you from getting the right dose of insulin.)

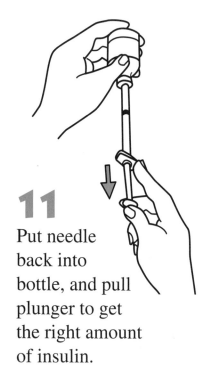

11

Put needle back into bottle, and pull plunger to get the right amount of insulin.

How to inject insulin with a syringe*

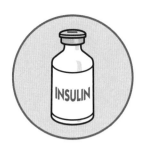

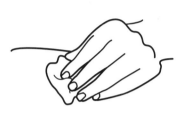

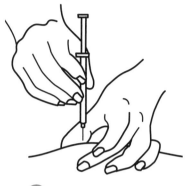

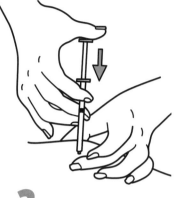

1
Follow your doctor's or diabetes educator's guidelines to clean the site. Either wipe with alcohol or wash with soap and water. Let area dry.

2
Hold syringe like a pencil. Pinch up the skin, and quickly push needle straight into your skin at a 90° angle. For sites with very little fat, check with your doctor or diabetes educator for special instructions.

3
Push plunger all the way down.

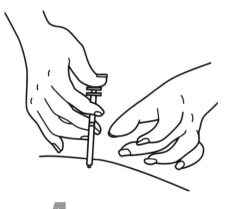

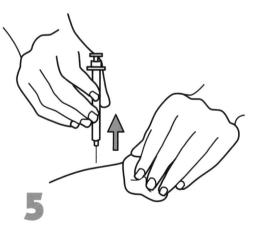

4
Let go of pinched skin.

5
Remove needle and syringe. Apply pressure to site.

Have extra insulin and syringes on hand at all times.

Keep supplies (syringes and insulin) in a clean, handy place.

*Check with your doctor or diabetes educator about how to use an insulin pen.

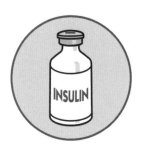

Mixing two kinds of insulin

If you need to inject 2 types of insulin (like short-acting and intermediate-acting), you may be able to mix them in one syringe. If they are mixed, they are injected at one time. To help you know which is which, the **intermediate (NPH) insulin is cloudy** and the **short-acting (regular) is clear.** Check with your doctor or diabetes educator to see if your insulins can be mixed. Do not mix Lantus insulin with any other insulin. Mixing will make it not effective.

Steps for mixing 2 types of insulins:

Prepare equipment the same as for single dose.

1 Roll intermediate (cloudy) insulin between hands to mix. Wipe the tops of both bottles with alcohol.

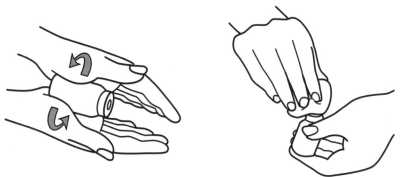

2 Into the intermediate (cloudy) bottle, inject air equal to the number of units you will be taking (for example, 20 units). Don't draw back the insulin yet. Remove the syringe.

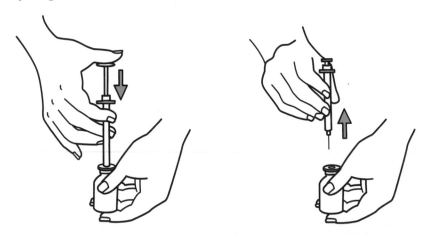

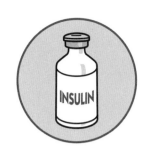

3 Next, inject air equal to your dose into the clear insulin (for example, short-acting, 5 units). Draw up the right insulin dose, and remove any bubbles.

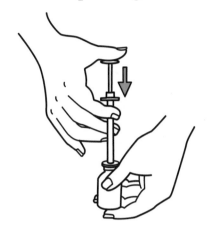
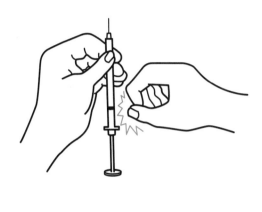

4 Insert needle back into cloudy insulin, and draw up dose (for example, 20 units). This means you will pull the plunger to 25 units since you already have 5 units in your syringe. Again, watch for air bubbles.

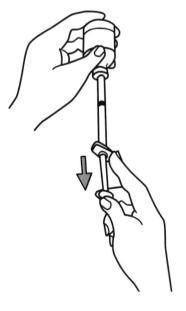

You are now ready to follow the injection steps on page 53.

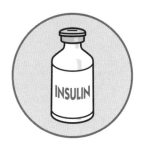

Insulin Pumps

For some, an insulin pump is an alternate for insulin delivery and may be the answer for better blood glucose control. A pump takes the place of insulin injections. But it does not take the place of regular blood glucose checks.

An insulin pump is about the size of a beeper. It delivers insulin through a thin plastic tube called an infusion set. There is a needle at the end that is inserted under the skin (most often in the abdomen).

A pump allows you to get a continuous amount of insulin (called a basal rate) over a 24-hour period. This insulin keeps blood glucose in check between meals and over night. When food is eaten, it allows a single large infusion (bolus) of insulin to match the amount of food that is eaten.

You and your doctor need to decide if a pump is right for you. But, before you decide, there are some things to keep in mind:

- the pump is expensive, so check with your insurance carrier to see if it is covered
- it takes a few months to get the doses right
- it can cause skin problems or infections
- the infusion line may clog or there may be other technical problems
- you have to change the infusion sets about every 2-3 days

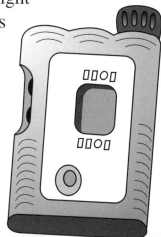

Benefits of the pump:

- better blood glucose control
- your schedule can be more flexible
- fewer insulin injections

Oral Agents

Medicines taken by mouth to lower blood glucose are called oral agents. **They are not insulin.** There are different types of these pills, and **each acts in a different way** to control blood glucose levels. Each oral agent acts in one of these ways:

- stimulates the pancreas to make more insulin

- slows the digestion of some carbohydrates

- keeps the liver from releasing too much glucose

- makes muscle cells more sensitive to insulin

These medicines may be used alone or combined. If they are prescribed for you, you must balance them with your meal planning and exercise. **It is important to take the right dose at the same time(s) each day.** Do not stop taking your medicine without the advice of your doctor or diabetes educator. Write in the name of your medicine(s) and the time(s) of day you take it:

Medicine name	Time taken	Amount taken

Be sure to discuss the side effects of your medicines and the best time to take them with your doctor or diabetes educator.

CAUTION: Alcohol and medicines (even over-the-counter) can affect the way some oral agents work. Be sure your doctor knows about all other medicines you take.

Knowing When You Are Balanced

You now know what the treatment of diabetes includes. But to know if your diet, exercise and use of insulin or pills (for some) are working, **you need to know your blood glucose level.** The best way to know this is by frequent blood tests. These tests can be done by anyone with diabetes. This includes women who only have diabetes during pregnancy. It is called **self-monitoring of blood glucose.**

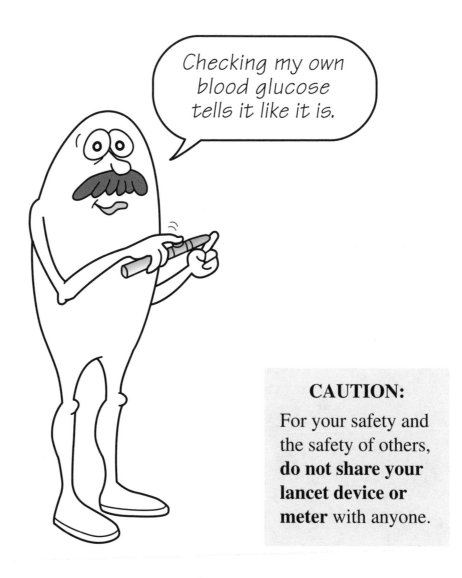

Checking my own blood glucose tells it like it is.

CAUTION:

For your safety and the safety of others, **do not share your lancet device or meter** with anyone.

Self-monitoring of Blood Glucose (SMBG)

Self-monitoring of your blood glucose can help you control your diabetes. From self-monitoring you find:

- your blood glucose level **at the moment** of testing

- how **food, exercise**, **medicines** and **illness** or **stress** affect blood glucose levels

- **early warning signs** of very low blood glucose (hypoglycemia—page 65)

- **early warning signs** of very high blood glucose (hyperglycemia—page 68)

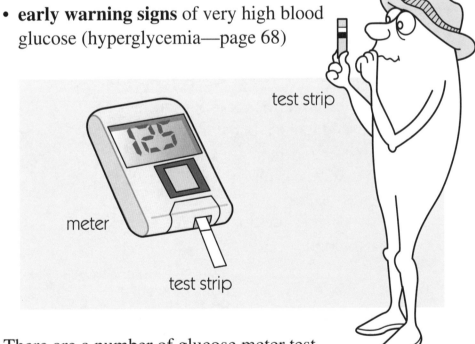

test strip

meter

test strip

There are a number of glucose meter test kits. Your doctor, nurse or diabetes educator will show you which to use and how. The blood tests are done with test strips alone or with test strips and a meter.

Insurance may cover the cost of many blood glucose test materials. Check to see what your insurance covers.

Testing

It is important to follow the instructions that come with your test kit to get a correct reading. For blood testing, you will need a drop of blood applied to the test strip.

1. First read the directions that came with your test kit.

2. Wash your hands with soap and warm water. If you select a site other than your hand, clean it with soap and water too.

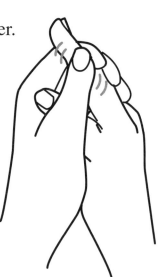

3. Rub or "milk" your finger. Do this a number of times to increase the flow of blood to the finger.

4. Follow the directions on your lancet device, and make a puncture on the side of a fingertip or site chosen. Use a new lancet for each stick.

5. Gently squeeze the finger to get a large drop of blood.

6. Apply the drop of blood onto the strip according to your test kit instructions. Do not rub or dab, it will be absorbed.

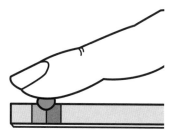

7. Go on with the test as directed.

8. Wait the correct amount of time, then read the test result at once and record it in your blood glucose records.

Blood Glucose Records

Frequent tests of your blood glucose provide important facts about your treatment plan. By keeping records of the test results, you and your doctor can better talk about any changes in your treatment that may improve control of your diabetes. This sample record might be helpful.

Review it with your doctor or diabetes educator to find **patterns.** An example of a pattern is high blood glucose every morning for several days. Your doctor or diabetes educator can work with you to find ways to improve patterns that are too high or too low for your blood glucose target range.

DATE	BREAKFAST		LUNCH		DINNER		BEDTIME		COMMENTS
	blood glucose	insulin/ oral agent	blood glucose	insulin/ oral agent	blood glucose	insulin/ oral agent	blood glucose	insulin/ oral agent	Food, exercise, ketones, stress, general health

A Test To Check On Long-Term Control

There is a test that can tell you if blood glucose is close to normal (or not) over a period of time. The test is called **Hemoglobin A1c.** Other names for it are:

- **"HgbA1c" or "A1c"**
- **Glycosylated Hemoglobin**
- **Glycohemoglobin**

Red blood cells contain a protein called hemoglobin. When glucose comes into contact with hemoglobin, it stays there for the life of the red blood cell. The combined hemoglobin and glucose is called Hemoglobin A1c (HgbA1c). The level of HgbA1c shows an average blood glucose over the last 2 or 3 months.

The American Association of Clinical Endocrinologists recommends a HgbA1c **goal of less than 6.5%** for adult men and non-pregnant women. Different goals may be set for women during pregnancy or for children. In a person who does not have diabetes, HgbA1c is most often 4–6%. People with diabetes should try to get levels as close to normal as they can by following their treatment plans. People with diabetes should have this test done at least twice a year.

Ask your doctor about this test. It's one more way that you can make sure your treatment plan is working.

Always know your HgbA1c score.

My score is _____.

Testing For Ketones

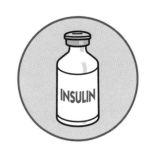

(for those taking insulin)

The body must have glucose for energy. When it can't get enough glucose from the foods you eat, it breaks down stored fat,* and ketones are formed. This causes a dangerous condition called ketoacidosis. If not treated, this can lead to coma and/or death.

Keep test materials on hand, and test for ketones when these occur:

- You just found out you have diabetes and are **still learning to balance your treatment.**

- **You have symptoms of high blood glucose.** (See page 68.)

- You test your blood, and **blood glucose is 240 or higher.**

- **You are sick or have an infection.** (This is most true if you are vomiting or have diarrhea and are losing body fluids.)

- **You are pregnant.** During pregnancy you may be asked to check for ketones more often and for a lower blood glucose result. Check with your doctor.

This does not refer to fatty buildup such as cholesterol.

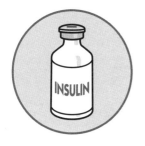

Ketones can be tested in urine or blood. However, it is done more frequently in urine. There are several products you can buy for this test.

- **Follow package directions carefully.** Don't use urine test materials after their expiration date.

- Store urine test materials **away from sunlight, heat and moisture.**

Call your doctor at once if you have blood glucose over the top of your range and ketones.

To test ketones in blood, follow meter instructions.

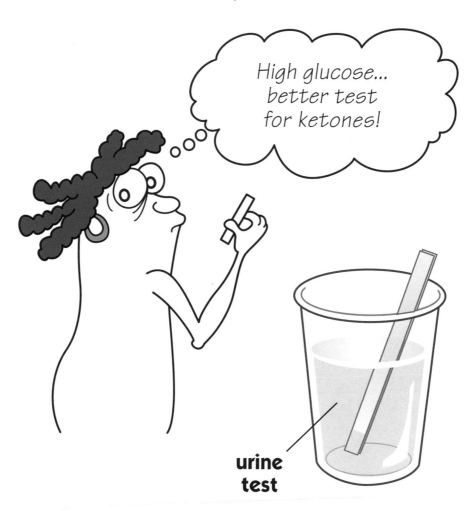

High glucose... better test for ketones!

urine test

Knowing When You Are Out Of Balance

Low Blood Glucose

For people who take insulin or pills for diabetes, there may be times when you have low blood glucose (hypoglycemia). If you have low blood glucose, you may have **one or more of these symptoms:**

early stage	*later*
shaky	slurred speech
sweaty	staggering
headache	confusion
hungry	convulsions
dizzy	unconsciousness
fast heartbeat	agressiveness
irritable/moody	
numbness around mouth/lips	
tingling	

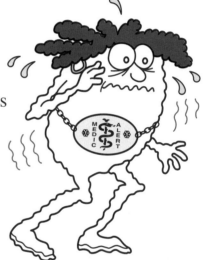

Some people don't notice these symptoms right away. For this reason, those close to you (family, friends, teachers, coaches, etc.) should know the symptoms of low blood glucose and how to treat them. Often the change from the early to the later stage is so fast that someone else must give proper treatment. For this reason, **always wear ID.**

The lowest safe blood glucose for me is:

_____

If you think your blood glucose is low, test it or have someone test it for you. A blood glucose of 70 or less is considered low for men and non-pregnant women with diabetes who are taking insulin or oral agents that can cause low blood glucose. **If you think your blood glucose is low** and you cannot test it, **always treat the symptoms.**

Causes of low blood glucose:
- too much insulin or oral medicine
- too little food (skipped or delayed meals)
- a lot of exercise without extra food

Preventing low blood glucose:
- Take the correct amount of medication (insulin or pills).
- Never skip or delay meals.
- Space meals 4–5 hours apart.
- Eat your scheduled snacks as needed.
- Test blood glucose regularly. Look for patterns of low blood glucose and discuss with your doctor.
- If on insulin, learn to relate low blood glucose to your exercise, peak action of insulin and meals.
- Always carry a good sugar source (glucose tablets).

Treatment for low blood glucose (Treat at once!)

Step 1: Test your blood glucose level (if possible). If it is 70 or less, eat or drink one of these:
- ½ cup fruit juice or ½ can regular soda (not diet)
- 1 tablespoon of sugar or 4 sugar cubes
- 6–7 hard candies (like Lifesavers)
- 2 tsp molasses, corn syrup or honey
- glucose tablets (take 3–4 tablets) available over-the-counter

NOTE: When you feel well again, think about what may have caused this reaction so you can prevent it in the future.

Step 2: Wait 15 minutes and retest. If it is still less than 70, or you still have symptoms, repeat Step 1 and 2 until you reach 70 or more.

Step 3: Once your blood glucose is above 70, you need to eat something. If your next meal is not scheduled for more than an hour, eat a snack (such as cheese/cracker/milk).

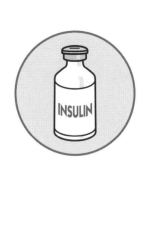

Glucagon* may be used for severe hypoglycemia when a person passes out or cannot swallow. It is sold by prescription in a kit with a filled syringe and a bottle of powder that must be mixed. Follow the directions for mixing the glucagon then inject it as you would insulin. A family member or friend needs to know how to do this and may also need to call for emergency assistance.

Glucagon Emergency Kit

1. Remove caps from powder bottle and syringe.

2. Insert needle into bottle and inject liquid. (Remove syringe from bottle. Keep needle sterile.)

3. **Shake bottle until liquid and powder mix.**

4. Draw up mixture and remove syringe.

5. Inject contents of syringe into any area used for insulin injections.

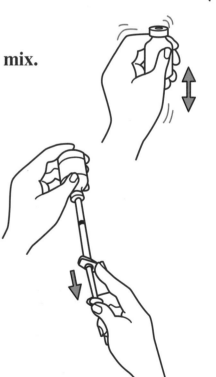

Be sure the person is placed on his side or stomach in case he vomits.

After injection, a person should respond in 10–15 minutes. He should eat a snack at this time. (Good choices are a small meat sandwich, milk, or peanut butter and crackers.) **Call the doctor after using glucagon.**

Be prepared if you take insulin. Ask your doctor for a glucagon kit, keep it on hand and teach someone else how to use it, too.

Glucagon is a hormone made by the pancreas, but it has the opposite effect of insulin. Glucagon raises blood glucose.

High Blood Glucose

Whether you inject insulin or not, you may have high blood glucose at some time. This is called *hyperglycemia*. If you have Type 1 diabetes, high blood glucose could lead to ketoacidosis or coma. It rarely leads to this if you have Type 2 diabetes, but it can. Whether you have Type 1 or Type 2 diabetes, over time, high blood glucose can damage your body organs.

When blood glucose is high, you may have one or more of these symptoms:

early stage	*later*
thirst (dry mouth)	nausea, vomiting
frequent urination	stomach cramps
blurred vision	sweet, fruity breath
feeling tired	flushed skin
itching (vaginal/genital)	deep, rapid breathing
	unconsciousness
	death (if not treated)

Glucose might be high. Better check it now.

Someone close to you should know these symptoms and how to treat them.

Causes of high blood glucose:

- skipped insulin injections or not taking right amount
- not taking the right amount of oral agents
- illness or infection
- severe stress or trauma (surgery, accident, etc.)
- overeating
- eating concentrated sweets
- insulin that has expired or has been damaged by heat or cold

Preventing high blood glucose:

- If on insulin, inject the right amount at the right times each day.
- Test your blood glucose regularly.
- See a doctor when ill or if you have an infection.
- Discuss a sick day plan with your doctor.
- Test your urine for ketones when glucose is high or when you are sick, and report this to your doctor.
- Follow your meal plan.
- Do not exercise if your blood glucose is very high (240+) or ketones are present. (Exercise at this time can make blood glucose go even higher.)

Treatment for high blood glucose:

- Test your blood for glucose and urine for ketones.
- If your blood glucose is high (240+) and your urine shows ketones, call in the results of these tests to your doctor **right away**. You may need to be in the hospital or to take extra fast-acting insulin.
- Drink plenty of sugar-free fluids.

Illness Or Infection

Illness or infection can throw your diabetes out of control. Know what to do when this happens. If not treated quickly, illness or infection can cause high blood glucose and ketones and lead to ketoacidosis and coma. Here are some tips to keep you out of trouble:

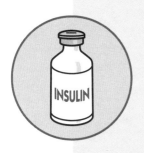

- **Take insulin every day** (if prescribed), **whether sick or well.**

- **More fast-acting insulin may be needed when you're ill.** Call your doctor if you:
  - vomit more than once
  - have diarrhea more than 5 times
  - are ill for more than 24 hours
  - can't keep food or drinks down

- **Check your blood glucose more often and test urine for ketones.** High blood glucose and ketones are major warning signs. Call your doctor if they are high.

- **Drink extra fluids** if you have diarrhea or are vomiting. If you're sick to your stomach, suck on ice chips.

- **If you can't eat your usual meal plan,** drink clear broths, unsweetened juices, bouillon or tea. Often Jell-O, dry toast or crackers will stay down. A "sick day diet" can be worked out for you by a registered dietitian.

- **If you can't eat solid foods,** take sips of ginger ale or a cola to meet your carbohydrates need.* You will need 50 g of carbohydrate for each meal missed. For example: 12 oz of ginger ale = 30 g; 12 oz of cola = 40 g.

drinks with real sugar, not diet drinks.

• **Call your doctor if you can't eat or drink anything without getting sick to your stomach.** If you are this sick, be sure to test (or have someone test) your blood for glucose and urine for ketones. Your doctor will want to know your blood glucose level and if ketones are present in your urine. If you can't keep food or fluids down for more than 4 hours, call your doctor.

Illness or infection puts a strain on balance!

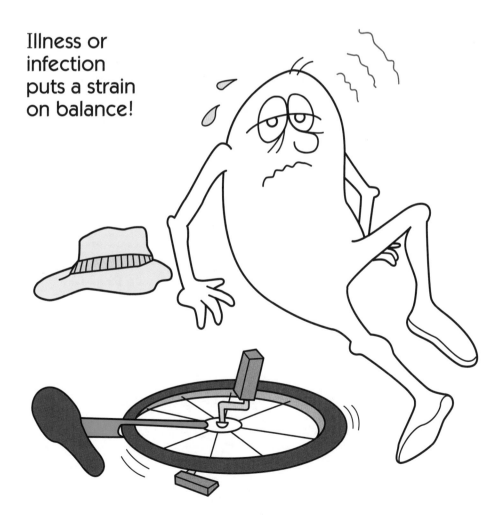

Diabetes Affects The Whole Body

It is likely that you know some of the complications of diabetes. Maybe you know someone who lost a leg or his eyesight because of this disease.

It is true that diabetes is serious, especially if not controlled. It is also true that even if you are in good control, you may still have problems. But if you take care of yourself as well as you can, chances are very good that you may prevent or reduce these risks.

The next section tells you about the complications of diabetes and gives tips on taking good care of your body.

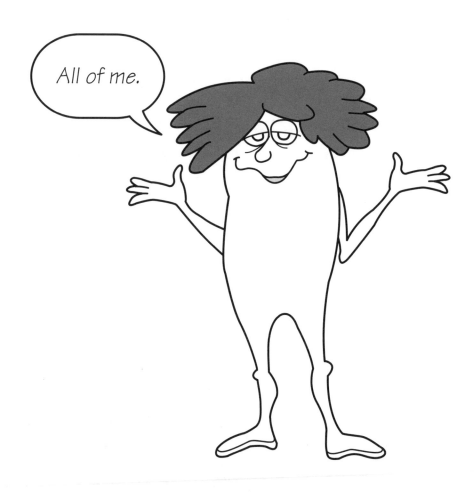

All of me.

Heart & Blood Vessels

Having diabetes can increase your chances for high blood pressure, heart disease or stroke. These are the leading cause of death in people with diabetes. But many of the things you do to control diabetes can also help your heart and blood vessels.

These are ways to help:

- If you smoke, quit. Smoking is the worst thing you can do for your heart. It raises blood pressure, tightens blood vessels and leads to fatty buildup in your arteries.

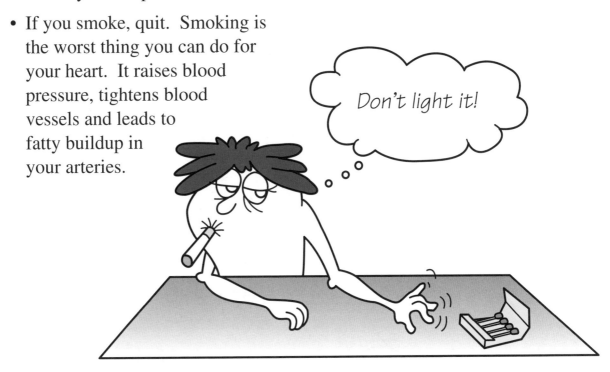

- Maintain a healthy weight.

- Eat a low-fat diet.

- Control blood pressure. High blood pressure can lead to heart disease, kidney failure and eye problems. Your blood pressure should be less than 130/80.

- Control blood cholesterol and fats.

- Exercise regularly.

- Ask your doctor about daily aspirin therapy to prevent heart and blood vessel disease.

Kidneys

Kidney disease (nephropathy) or renal failure is another risk for people with diabetes. Your risk for it goes up with the number of years you have had diabetes. It also increases if you have high blood pressure and frequent urinary tract infections.

Kidney disease is very sneaky. A person can lose 70% of kidney function and not know it. Then when it is finally found, the kidneys are already damaged. Again, control and prevention will be your best protection.

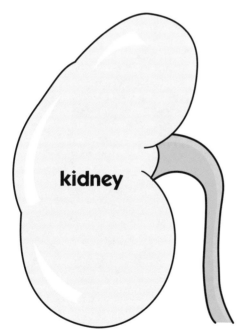

- Have a **microalbumin urine test** at least once a year to check for protein in the urine.

- **Call your doctor** at the first sign of a urinary tract infection.* This needs to be treated right away.

- Keep blood glucose and blood pressure **as normal as possible.**

- **Talk with your diabetes doctor before having any tests where dyes are used.**

- **See a nephrologist at the first sign of microalbumin.**

*blood or pus in urine; burning with urination and/or frequent urination

Eyes

Over a period of years, high blood glucose can cause changes in the retina* and small blood vessels of the eye (retinopathy). This affects over 50% of the people who have had diabetes more than 10 years, making diabetes a leading cause of blindness. Why it happens to some people and not others may be due to:

- **the age** at which a person got diabetes

- **how many years** a person has had diabetes

- blood glucose **control**

- if a person also has **high blood pressure** (hypertension)

- increased risk during pregnancy

Most cases of blindness and other eye problems (cataracts, glaucoma) can be prevented with regular treatment. **You should have your eyes dilated and examined once a year.** Report any vision changes to your eye doctor right away. Keep blood glucose down, and control high blood pressure if you have it.

retina

*the layer of the eye which receives an image from the lens and sends it to the brain

Feet & Legs

People with diabetes need to take very good care of their feet and legs. There are 2 good reasons for doing this: poor circulation (vascular disease) and nerve damage (diabetic neuropathy).

Poor circulation (reduced blood flow) occurs when blood vessels leading to the feet and legs become narrow or harden. This is part of aging, but it often happens sooner in people with diabetes. When this happens, the legs and feet do not get enough white blood cells to fight infection. If not treated with care, simple cuts and sores can become serious ulcers and infections. These can lead to gangrene or amputation.

Nerve damage (neuropathy) is another complication of diabetes. It is most often related to how long a person has had diabetes and how well blood glucose has been controlled. It can affect many areas of the body such as the bladder, bowel and other organs. More often, it affects the feet and legs. The symptoms can be burning, aching, feel like "pins and needles" or loss of feeling. All of these range from mild to severe. The discomfort is often worse at night. With time and good blood glucose control, some of the damage can be reversed, but some can't. Balancing your act is the best defense.

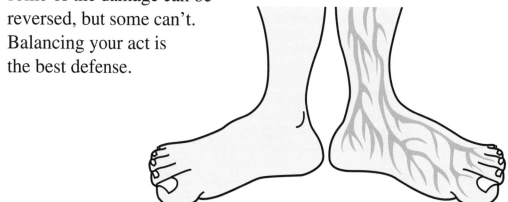

To improve blood flow to feet and legs:

- **Don't smoke.** Ask your doctor or diabetes educator for help quitting if you need it.

- **Control blood glucose and blood pressure.**

- **Exercise** regularly.

- **Sit with uncrossed legs,** and walk around during the day if you have a desk job.

- Wear shoes that fit well with plenty of room for your toes.

- **Do not wear** hose or socks with tight, elastic tops. Do not twist hose around legs to keep them up.

- Gently **massage cold feet.** Wear socks to bed if your feet stay cold.

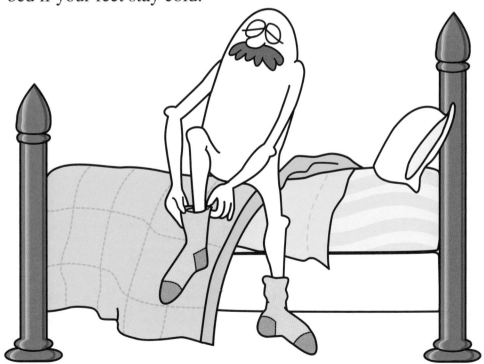

Do these for good foot care:

- **Check your feet daily** for corns, callouses, blisters, cuts, scrapes, bruises or infections. If you have any of these, see your doctor or a podiatrist. Don't treat foot problems yourself.

  - Check in good light.
  - If you wear glasses, put them on.
  - Use a mirror to help see the bottom of your feet.
  - If you can't bend over to check your feet, ask someone to check for you.

- **Wash feet** gently each day. (But **do not soak** feet.)

- Have your doctor or podiatrist show you how to file (with an emery board) or trim your toenails. **File or trim nails just after bathing** when they are soft.

- If your feet are **dry and scaly,** rub on a mild lotion (but not between toes) before bedtime.

- Have a **"socks off" exam** at each visit to your doctor.

- **Do not go barefoot** (even to the bathroom at night).

- Wear shoes that **support** your feet and are **comfortable.** Break in new shoes slowly.

- Check inside your shoes for **torn linings** or **things that don't belong** (like a stone).

- **To avoid a burn,** test bath water with your elbow or hand. Your feet may be too numb to feel the heat. And **never use a heating pad** on your feet or legs.

Skin

Since people with diabetes may have poor blood flow, care of the skin is important.

- Wear a wide-brimmed hat and use sunscreen to prevent sunburn.

- Keep your skin clean.

- Use a moisturizer to keep skin from getting too dry.

- Tell your doctor if you have redness, swelling or pain for more than one day.

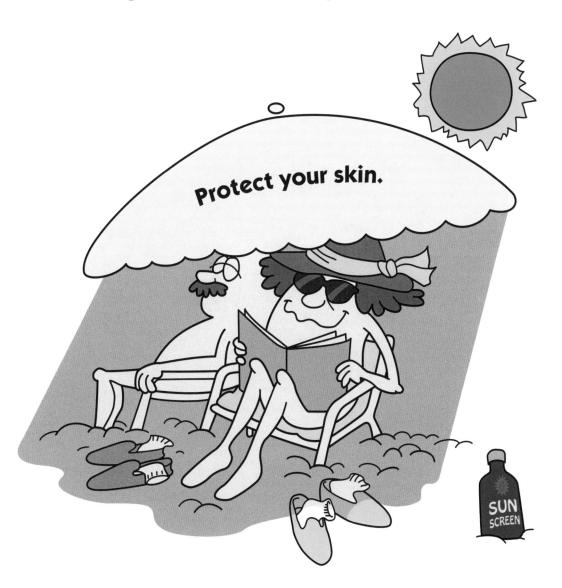

Protect your skin.

Teeth & Gums

Diabetes may make you more prone to gum disease. As people age, it is most often gum disease, not tooth decay, that causes loss of teeth. Be sure to do these:

- Have **regular checkups** with your dentist every 6 months.

- Be sure to **tell your dentist** you have diabetes.

- **Clean and floss** your teeth daily.

Your dentist can tell you how to care for your teeth and gums.

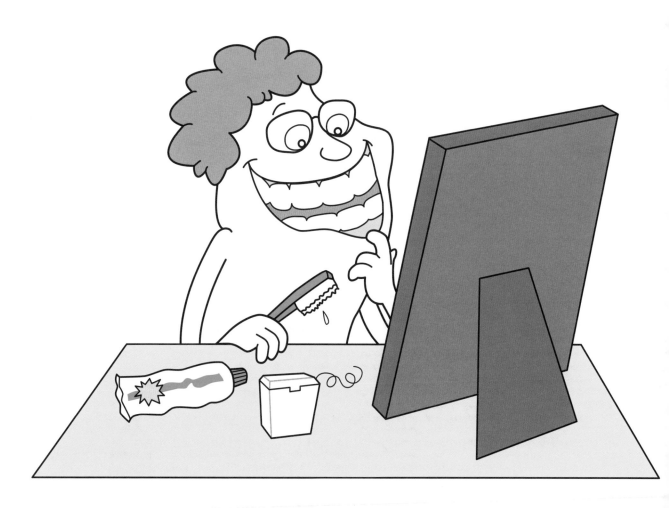

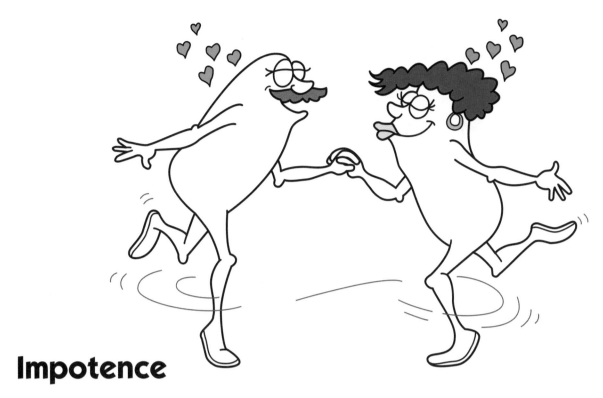

Impotence

Staying in balance promotes a healthier, sexier you.

High blood glucose (over a long time) can lead to loss of nerve function and poor blood flow. This may show up as impotence in men. Sometimes, impotence is a side effect of medicine (ex., drugs taken to control high blood pressure). It can also be due to hormones or a psychological problem. Other times, impotence is a short-term problem caused by short, uncontrolled periods of high blood glucose.

These days there's a lot that can be done for this problem. There are many ways to help sexual function, including medicines and penile implants. Your doctor can help you get the right answer for you.

For women, it is thought that long periods of high blood glucose can cause reduced vaginal fluids and lead to loss of orgasm. There are special vaginal lubricants to help with this. Ask your doctor. It is known that high blood glucose can lead to frequent vaginal infections which must be treated.

Stress and Depression

Learning that you have diabetes can be stressful. Having diabetes means making changes to your lifestyle. And making changes can lead to stress. Too much stress can cause the body to release stored glucose. This can raise your blood glucose levels, which makes it harder to control diabetes.

Knowing that you have to "manage" a condition for the rest of your life can also be stressful. Being stressed out for a long period of time can lead to you being sad, angry or depressed.

If you feel stressed because of diabetes, you are not alone. But it's up to you to do something about it. Having a positive outlook, learning about diabetes and taking control of managing it will help you through the stressful times. You can also:

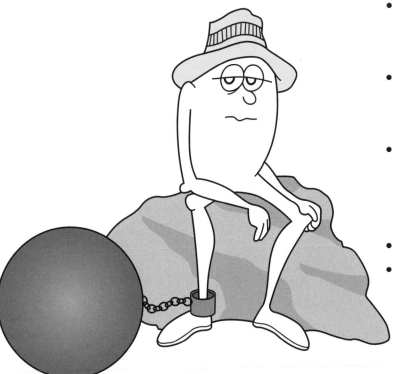

- find a support group with others who have diabetes
- talk with a friend or family member about how you feel
- have a positive attitude about yourself, your life and those around you
- learn to relax
- get more active

Other Things To Consider When You Have Diabetes

Identification (ID)

Wear some kind of ID* at all times. There are nice bracelets or necklaces for this purpose. ID lets others know you have diabetes if you can't tell them yourself (if you are unconscious, injured or are acting strangely due to low blood glucose). The right treatment can then be given.

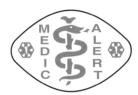

Front

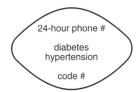

24-hour phone #

diabetes
hypertension

code #

Back

* *Medic Alert is one type of ID you can buy. You can get either a bracelet or necklace. On this ID you will have a 24-hour emergency number, a list of your medical conditions and a code number assigned to you when the bracelet is bought. Your medical records are stored by this code number. Information about these bracelets can be ordered from:*

MedicAlert Foundation
2323 Colorado Ave., Turlock, CA 95382
1-888-633-4298 • www.medicalert.org

Insurance

People with diabetes can get health and life insurance. As for anyone, the younger you are when you buy insurance, the better. Your premiums may be slightly higher, but insurers will vary costs according to:

- **how long you've had diabetes**
- **how well it is controlled**
- **complications, if any**

Also, insurance companies may want to ask your doctor about your diabetes.

Employment

By law, you can't be discriminated against for most jobs because of your diabetes. The Americans With Disabilities Act makes sure employers have fair hiring customs.

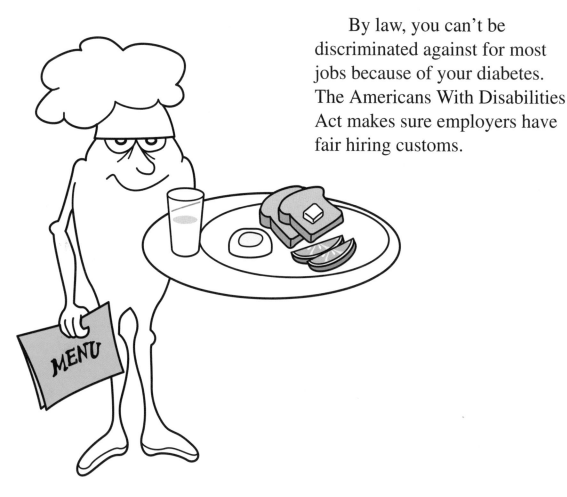

Travel

Whether on the road for an hour or a number of weeks, you need to plan ahead. Check with your doctor or diabetes educator before traveling for important tips on staying in control. Be sure to ask about:

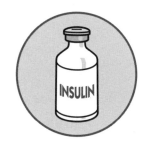

- meal planning

- how often to test your blood glucose

- what to do in case of illness or injury

- medicines

When traveling by car, stop for meals or snacks at the proper times. Stop just to rest and stretch. Carry juice, crackers and/or food in your car in case of low blood glucose and traffic delays. If you are driving, always check your blood glucose before starting and every 2 hours. It must be at least 100.

When traveling by plane, you have to consider time changes. If you don't know how to adjust your meals and insulin for this, ask your doctor or diabetes educator for help. Special meals may be ordered ahead of time from the airline. Carry some food with you in case of delays.

Also, **carry all diabetes supplies, medicines and food with you on the plane** in case luggage is lost or delayed. (See page 48 for tips on insulin storage.)

If traveling to a **foreign country,** it is safer to carry your own diabetes medicines and supplies. Be sure to **carry a brief medical record and a signed statement from your doctor that says you take insulin.** This may save delay and embarrassment when going through customs and with security issues.

Finally, **always wear an ID tag or bracelet and comfortable shoes.**

CAUTION

Some insulin and syringes in foreign countries are not U-100. Make sure to check what type of insulin and syringe you buy before you use it. Diabetes supplies may have a different name in other countries.

Special Concerns For Women With Diabetes

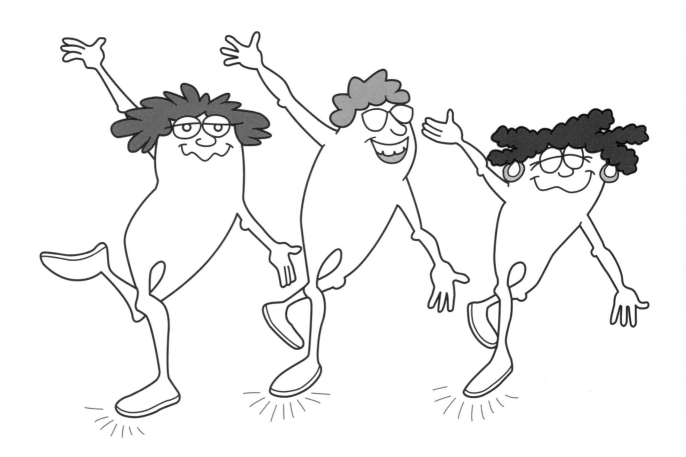

Menstrual Periods & Menopause

Changes in hormone levels can cause swings of high or low blood glucose. So you may need to check your blood glucose levels and your urine for ketones more often right before and during menstrual periods or menopause.

Pregnancy

If you have diabetes and plan to become pregnant, first talk to your doctor. You will need to be in very good control **before** you decide to become pregnant. Getting pregnant while your diabetes is out of control can result in birth defects.

If you don't want to become pregnant, talk with your doctor about birth control.

Women on pills for diabetes should see their doctor before becoming pregnant. Insulin is the only drug for diabetes approved by the FDA for pregnant women. Also, some pills to treat high blood pressure cannot be used safely during pregnancy. Your doctor will change you to medicines safe for you and your baby.

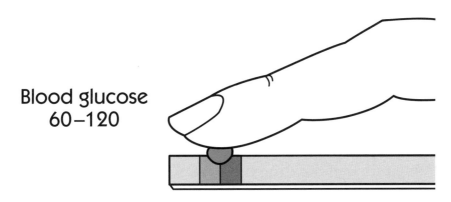

Blood glucose
60–120

More attention during pregnancy by the whole health care team will help you have a healthy baby. **Frequent self-monitoring of blood glucose** is the best way to see if your blood glucose is controlled. A healthy blood glucose range while you are pregnant is usually 60–120. Your HgbA1c should also be less than 6.5%. (See page 62.) If you maintain good control and keep scheduled visits with your health care team, your chances for having a delivery without problems and a healthy baby are excellent.

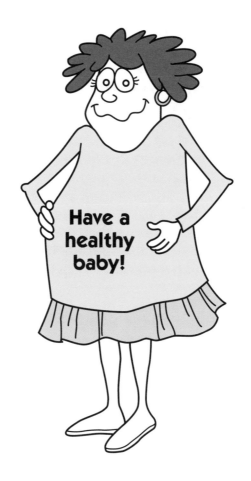

Some women get diabetes when they are pregnant. This is called **gestational diabetes mellitus** (GDM). Most often it is found during the 24–28th week of pregnancy, and can often be managed with meal planning. Insulin may be needed to control blood glucose in some pregnant women. Most of the time gestational diabetes goes away after the baby is born. (It would be wise, though, to be checked for high blood glucose at the 6-week checkup, at 6 months after delivery and from time to time thereafter. You may be prone to diabetes later in life, especially if you are overweight.)

What's New

When you see how far we have come in diabetes control, you can be excited about the future.

- **Improved insulins** (analogs) are available.

- **New oral agents** (drugs) for diabetes are available.

- **Alternate routes** for insulin are being tested.

- **Blood glucose testing** is easier each year. Continuous "no-stick" or less-invasive methods are now being tested and approved.

- New drugs are being made that **limit the complications** of diabetes.

- **Islet cell* transplants** are being tested and will most likely be improved.

- **New uses for certain drugs** are being found to keep insulin-producing cells from being destroyed and to reduce kidney damage.

- **Closed loop insulin pump** is being developed as an artificial pancreas.

- A vaccine for Type 1 diabetes is being tested.

Until a cure for diabetes is found, learn as much as you can about it. Work hard to control it. We hope this book helped you get started.

cells from the pancreas

Appendix

The next pages list a few of the many books, magazines and newsletters for people with diabetes. Two pages on alcohol give you facts about this drug and list the exchange values of many drinks. There is also a page provided for meal planning.

Each year there are new materials and products for the control of diabetes. If you subscribe to *Diabetes Forecast* or *Diabetes Self-Management* (page 92), you will see many ads for these.

Books

Order from:
Pritchett & Hull Assoc.
Suite 110
3440 Oakcliff Rd., NE
Atlanta, GA 30340:

Balance Your Food Act
(a food book for adults with diabetes) Explains the benefits of meal planning in diabetes control. Use along with the advice of your doctor and dietitian.

Order from other publishers
or major bookstores:

World-Class Diabetic Cooking
Order from:
American Diabetes Association
1701 N. Beaureguard Street
Alexandria, VA 22311
(800) Diabetes (342-2383)
(Request a catalog of their other diabetes cookbooks and materials.)

The All-New Diabetic Cookbook
Order from:
Nelson Direct
P.O. Box 140300
Nashville, TN 37214-0300
(800) 441-0511
www.rutledgehillpress.com

The Diabetic Gourmet
Order from:
Diabetes Self-Management
DSM Books
P.O. Box 11066
Des Moines, IA 50336-1066
(800) 664-9269
www.diabetes-self-mgmt.com

Magazines & Newsletters

Diabetes Forecast
MAGAZINE: monthly
(Sent to members of the
American Diabetes Association)
American Diabetes Association
1701 N. Beaureguard Street
Alexandria, VA 22311

(800) 806-7801
www.diabetes.org/publications

Diabetes Self-Management
MAGAZINE: 6 issues a yr.
Order from:
Diabetes Self-Management
Subscription Services
P.O. Box 52890
Boulder, CO 80322

(800) 234-0923
www.diabetes-self-mgmt.com

Diabetes Interview
MAGAZINE: monthly
(800) 234-1218
www.diabetesworld.com

Exchange Lists

The **Exchange Lists
for Meal Planning** can
be ordered from:
American Diabetes Association
1701 N. Beaureguard Street
Alexandria, VA 22311
(800) Diabetes (342-2383)
www.diabetes.org

Good Health Eating Guide
(Canadian Exchange List)
Order from:
Canadian Diabetes Association
National Office
15 Toronto Street, Suite 800
Toronto, Ontario
Canada M5C2E3

(800) BANTING
(416) 363-3373
www.diabetes.ca

American Dietetic Association
120 South Riverside Plaza,
Suite 2000
Chicago, IL 60606-6995

(800) 877-1600

www.eatright.org

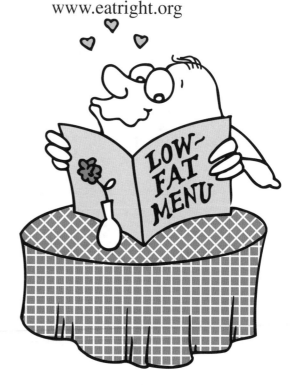

National Offices Of Associations & Foundations

American Association of Diabetes Educators
(for names of diabetes educators in your area)
100 West Monroe Street,
Suite 400
Chicago, IL 60603
(800) 338-3633
www.aadenet.org

American Diabetes Association
1701 N. Beaureguard Street
Alexandria, VA 22311
(800) 232-3472
www.diabetes.org

American Dietetic Association
120 South Riverside Plaza,
Suite 2000
Chicago, IL 60606-6995
(800) 877-1600
www.eatright.org

Canadian Diabetes Association
National Office
15 Toronto Street, Suite 800
Toronto, Ontario
Canada M5C 2E3
(800) BANTING
(416) 363-3373
www.diabetes.ca

National Diabetes Information Clearinghouse
1 Information Way
Bethesda, MD 20892-3560
(301) 654-3327
www.niddk.nih.gov

Juvenile Diabetes Research Foundation
120 Wall Street
New York, NY 10005-4001
1-800-533-CURE (2873)
www.jdrf.org

Other addresses or phone #'s important to me:

Doctor:_____

Diabetes nurse: _____

Dietitian: _____

Pharmacist: _____

Products I use: _____

Meal Planning

Your nurse or dietitian can help you fill in this sample meal plan for _____ calories per day.

	Day 1	Day 2	Day 3
	Breakfast	*Breakfast*	*Breakfast*

____ **Carbohydrates:**
___ starch/bread .
___ fruit . . . .
___ vegetable. . . .
___ milk . . . .
____ **Meats** . . . .
____ **Fats** . . . .
____ **Free Foods** . . . .

	Lunch	*Lunch*	*Lunch*

____ **Carbohydrates:**
___ starch/bread .
___ fruit . . . .
___ vegetable. . . .
___ milk . . . .
____ **Meats** . . . .
____ **Fats** . . . .
____ **Free Foods** . . . .

	Supper	*Supper*	*Supper*

____ **Carbohydrates:**
___ starch/bread .
___ fruit . . . .
___ vegetable. . . .
___ milk . . . .
____ **Meats** . . . .
____ **Fats** . . . .
____ **Free Foods** . . . .

	Snack	*Snack*	*Snack*

____ **Carbohydrates:**
___ starch/bread .
___ fruit . . . .
___ vegetable. . . .
___ milk . . . .
____ **Meats** . . . .
____ **Fats** . . . .
____ **Free Foods** . . . .

Alcohol

You may be able to have alcohol in your diet, but **first ask your doctor.** A rule of thumb is to "be moderate." For women this means no more than 1 drink a day, (for men no more than 2 drinks a day) of the following: $1^1/_4$ oz liquor, 4 oz dry wine or 12 oz beer.

If your doctor says it's OK to drink alcohol, **meet with a dietitian or Certified Diabetes Educator** to review the use of alcohol in your meal plan. Here are some things to think about:

- Before you drink, your **diabetes should be well controlled.**

- Alcohol can cause problems with some oral medications.

- Alcohol has **calories but no nutrients.**

- **Eat just before you drink** or while drinking (never on an empty stomach), especially if insulin is peaking.

- Alcohol can **cause low blood glucose** and make it harder to know if you have an insulin reaction. If you are taking an **oral agent,** alcohol may cause some bad reactions (page 57).

- **Avoid very sweet drinks** like liqueurs and sweet wines or those made with tonic, soda pop, fruit juices, etc.

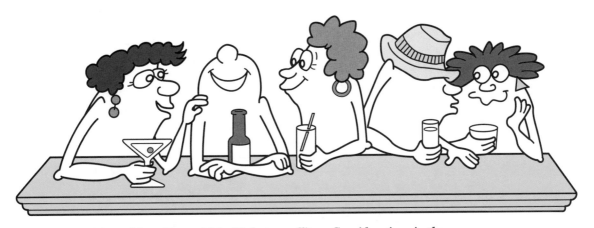

*Adapted from Franz, M.J.: **Diabetes mellitus: Considerations in the development of guidelines for the occasional use of alcohol.** © The American Dietetic Association. Reprinted by permission from JOURNAL OF THE AMERICAN DIETETIC ASSOCIATION, Vol. 83:147, 1983*

If Alcohol Is Allowed In Your Meal Plan

Item	Brand	Cal	Measure	Exchanges
Beer, ale (4.5% by volume)	Any	158	12 fl oz	1 carbohydrate, 2 fat
Brandy or cognac	Any	68	1 fl oz	1½ fat
Cider, fermented	Any	68	6 fl oz	1½ fat
Cordials: anisette, apricot brandy, Benedictine, creme de menthe, curacao	Any	79	⅔ fl oz	½ carbohydrate, 1 fat
Daiquiri	Any	124	3½ fl oz	½ carbohydrate, 2 fat
Gin, rum, scotch, vodka, whiskey	Any	135	1½ fl oz	3 fat
Manhattan	Any	169	3½ fl oz	½ carbohydrate, 3 fat
Martini	Any	135	3½ fl oz	3 fat
Old fashioned	Any	181	4 fl oz	½ carbohydrate, 3 fat
Port or muscatel	Any	158	3½ oz	1 carbohydrate, 2 fat
Tom Collins with regular mixer with artificial sweetener mixer	Any Any	192 158	10 fl oz 10 fl oz	½ carbohydrate, 3 fat 3½ fat
Sherry, dry	Any	85	2 fl oz	½ carbohydrate, 1 fat
Wine, dry table, 12% alcohol	‡	85	3½ fl oz	½ carbohydrate, 1 fat

‡*dry champagne, dry sauterne, chablis, claret,
  cabernet sauvignon, burgundy, etc.*

*Adapted from **Everything you always wanted to know about exchange values**,
Idaho Research Foundation, University of Idaho, Moscow, Idaho 83843.
Used with permission of the Foundation.*